THE HISTORY OF

Hair

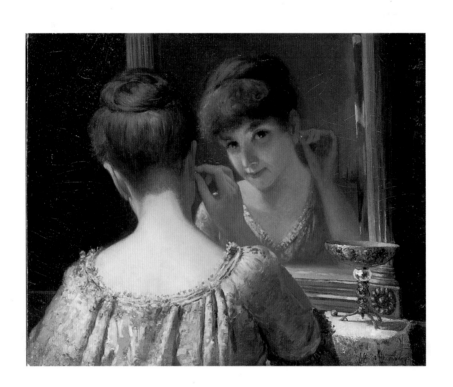

THE HISTORY OF

Hair

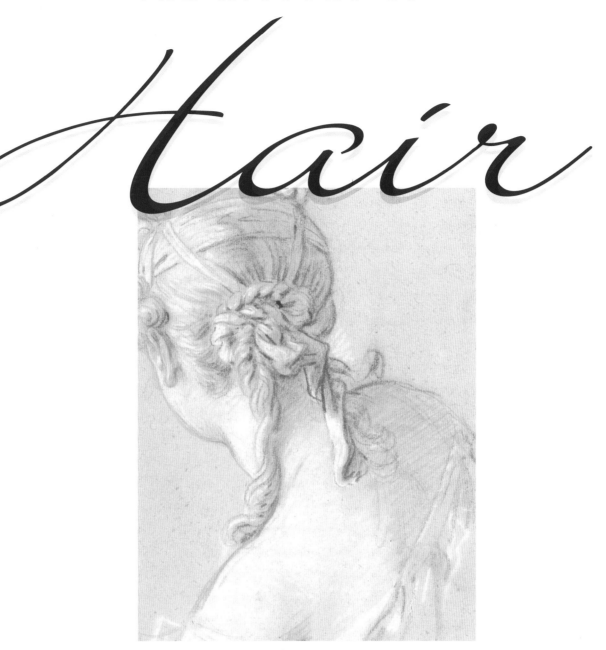

FASHION AND FANTASY DOWN THE AGES
Robin Bryer

Philip Wilson Publishers

for
JINKS
with love

First published in 2000 by
Philip Wilson Publishers
143-149 Great Portland Street
London W1W 6QN

Distributed in the USA and Canada by
Antique Collectors' Club
91 Market Street Industrial Park
Wappingers' Falls
New York 12590

Text © 2000 Robin Bryer

ISBN 0 85667 506 7

Edited by Helen Robertson
Designed by Keith & Clair Watson

Printed and bound in Italy by
Società Editoriale Lloyd, Srl, Trieste

CONTENTS

I HAVE ALWAYS BEEN FASCINATED BY HAIR. AS A SMALL BOY IN THE 'FIFTIES I WAS SENT ONCE A WEEK, ON MY BICYCLE, TO HAVE MY HAIR CUT. MR BOSWELL WOULD RUN HIS ELECTRIC CLIPPERS FIRMLY UP THE BACK AND SIDES OF MY HEAD BEFORE CLIPPING AWAY WITH HIS SCISSORS AT WHAT REMAINED ON TOP. FINALLY, AS HE SHOWED ME THE BACK OF MY HEAD IN HIS HAND MIRROR, HE WOULD ASK 'WOULD YOU LIKE SPRAY?' AND A CLOUD OF THIS WOULD BE APPLIED, WELDING MY PARTING IN PLACE.

ROBIN BRYER

What there was of my hair was mouse-coloured. Originally, it had been platinum blond. I used to look with wonder at a lock of it, saved from my first haircut, which my mother kept in a glass locket within a Victorian brooch designed to keep such special mementoes. Years later someone stole that brooch, and with it a part of me. It was made up of a gold filigree sprig of acorns within a circular gold frame; there was a glass door at the back, inside which nestled my hair. If you come across it, let me know.

The first night I spent away from home was with the family of a girl who had two pigtails. We played together in the loft above the stables and in the sandpit in the garden. I was fascinated by those rope-like pigtails, tied with ribbons at the end, and with the way she would toss one and then the other over her shoulders. I was likewise enthralled by the parting up the nape of her neck. We never mentioned those pigtails. They were just a part of her. I never saw her without them.

There was another small girl. She and I would explore the woods and sit in a hide waiting for badgers. Her hair was also long, and while the front was cut short in a fringe, it otherwise flowed freely and down her back. I was mortified, one Christmas, to find that it had been cut short to the shoulder. My father, with avuncular jocularity, gave her a bottle of hair restorer.

My mother had bobbed hair with a side parting and just two curls, one over each ear like earmuffs. She too had had long hair; there was a miniature of her as a small girl, painted on ivory. When she had it cut off, she had it made up into a tail of hair, bound at one end, like an old-fashioned fly whisk. My brother and I found it in the attic, wrapped in tissue paper. Delighted by our discovery, she tried to sell it, only to be told that, with the passing of the years, it was not in marketable condition. So, instead, we hung it up in a tree. For an entire spring, for miles around birds' nests were lined with our mother's hair.

My own hair is now as white as it was once blond. I wear it to the shoulder, putting to shame the wigs of judges when business takes me to the High Court. By contrast, the girls I played with as a child now have their hair cut 'sensibly' short.

Over the years I have discovered that I am not alone in my fascination with hair; it is almost universal. Indeed, it is an interest that artists through the ages have indulged in, vying with one another to catch hair's elusive qualities. Botticelli, Cranach, Renoir and Rossetti spring to mind as masters of painting hair. But not just they. Every portrait involves a painting of hair (or lack of it). When I look at a portrait, it is to the hair that I look first, and only then to the eyes and the mouth. The hair is as essential to the face as a frame is to a picture. Sometimes, the hair in a picture can be as difficult to capture as a fleeting smile on the lips of the sitter, so elusive are the colours glinting within it or the way it moves as the sitter moves. There are many commentaries on representations of faces in portraiture (David Piper's *The English Face* is perhaps the most memorable of these) as well as on costume as depicted in art. But nowhere could I find an informed account of hair down the ages, as conveyed by artists and cherished by their sitters and those who knew them – with the honourable exception of Richard Corson's scholarly and monumental *Fashions in Hair* with its comprehensive introduction both to primary sources and to anecdotal material.

What I felt urged to write was a personal commentary designed to complement rather than compete. Lecturing on Swan Hellenic cruises, I had quickly come to learn how fascinated an audience can become when one explores for them a universal but hitherto little-regarded avenue. I thought of calling the book 'Hair in Art', but my aim was to cover more than that. It was to record the significance of hair in our lives and in the lives of our ancestors. In the pages that lie ahead you will find that the attention is focused on the hair itself. You will be seeing old friends from an unfamiliar angle, in terms of both well-known pictures and their subjects. It is hair in all its fascinating convolutions, rather than the artists who painted it or the sitters whose hair it was, that is the focus of this book.

I have enjoyed combining my passion for hair with my love of paintings and people. To combine the three has been a very happy experience that I am now pleased to share with you.

THE UNIQUENESS OF HUMAN HAIR

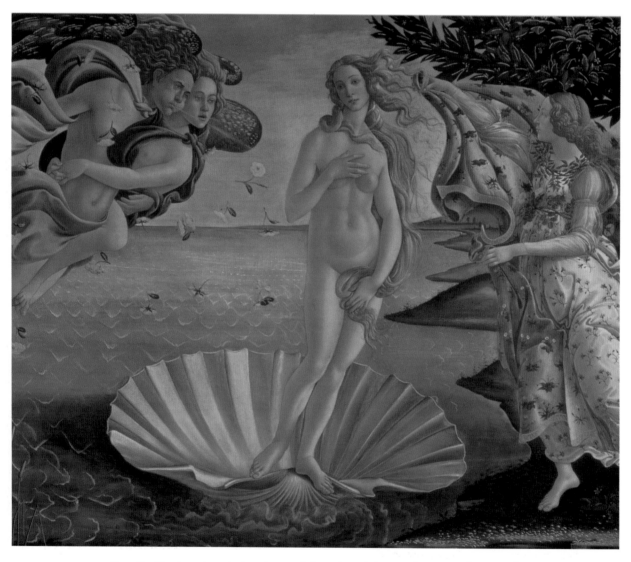

FIG. 1. The length and abundance of the subject's hair is the prime feature of
Botticelli's evocation of female beauty.
Sandro Botticelli, *The Birth of Venus* (detail), c.1485 (Galleria degli Uffizi, Florence)

Humans are unique in two aspects of their behaviour: wearing clothes and having their hair cut voluntarily. Botticelli's Venus (fig. 1) neither wears clothes nor has she submitted her hair to the scissors. Or has she? The tresses on either side of her head appear shorter than the long mane down her back, which she artfully holds forward with her left hand, while her right hand partly covers her breasts. The attendant to the right of her seems eager to clothe her, while the spirits to the left of her seem bent upon blowing her hair. She is, indeed, placed between nature and civilisation at this moment of birth. What is certain, however, is that it is her hair which is the most remarkable feature of Botticelli's embodiment of beauty.

Botticelli's Venus is born fully formed with abundant hair, whereas we know that many babies are born more or less bald. Hair comes later. It has its own birth. Indeed, it has a life of its own – that is, if something essentially dead can be said to have a life. It is only the root of the hair which is alive. The length of our hair, if we allow it to grow, is a record of the passing of time. Long hair is associated with young children; however, as hair grows at the rate of about six inches a year they must be a certain age to have long hair.

Whatever the biology of hair, it does seem to have a life that is independent of whoever it grows upon. One day it can be bad-tempered, another it can be good-tempered (hence the popular reference these days to having a 'good' or 'bad hair day'). It can be glossy or it can be listless. It can hang down, concealing the body. Then suddenly it can take on a life of its own, unveiling the body as it becomes a visual manifestation of that invisible phenomenon, a gust of wind. Indeed, quite as effectively as smoke in a scientist's wind tunnel, our hair can make wind strangely visible – and we a part of it, willingly or not – as it billows forward or backward from the head. When the wind blows, the long-haired are like full-rigged ships, sails billowing. The short-cropped are as undemonstrative as motor boats.

Movement is one characteristic of hair, colour is another. The colour of hair is invested with significance. Red hair grows more thickly and is associated with a fiery temper, but is that merely because it looks like

> ## Botticelli's Venus neither wears clothes nor has she submitted her hair to the scissors. Or has she?

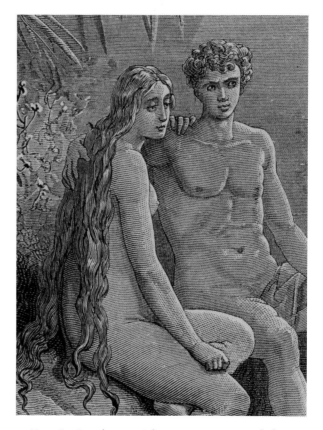

Fig. 2. Eve—but not Adam—as nature intended. A detail from Gustav Doré's illustration for Milton's *Paradise Lost.* (author's collection)

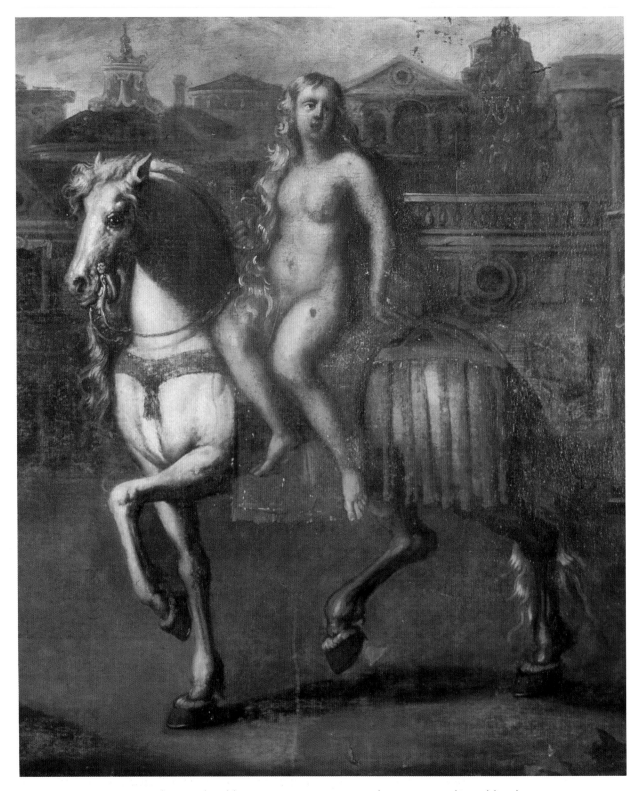

FIG. 3. Silver and gold — a mare's mane complements a girl's golden hair,
put to practical use here (famously) to maintain her modesty.
Flemish School, *Lady Godiva*, 1586 (Herbert Art Gallery & Museum, Coventry)

flames? Blond hair is associated with fun, or is that just because light shining on golden tresses brings a sense of happiness?

Dark hair has connotations of mystery and evil. The long black hair of the witch contrasts with the golden tresses of the fairy princess. Silver hair is a symbol of age and wisdom. However, as we shall see, these colour associations can change with the passage of time.

One long-held fallacy was that long hair is unique to womankind. The woman shares with the horse, the lion and the man the quality of having more hair on the head than on the body. She, however, is supposed to have still less hair on her body (ideally none at all)

Noel Coward once assured Eartha Kitt that not just on the head does hair continue to grow after death, but on the chest as well

but compensatingly more hair growing from her head. So it is that Eve is usually shown with an abundant head of hair falling to below her bottom but an entirely smooth body. Adam, by contrast, is typically depicted with short hair, a short beard and a relatively hairy body. If Eve is usually shown as nature intended, Adam most definitely is not, as in Gustav Doré's depiction where he is both short haired and without a beard (fig. 2).

Germaine Greer in *The Female Eunuch*, that quintessential book on feminism, notes that the assumption that women grow more hair on their heads than men is almost universal. She cites Bichat, who, writing as recently as 1846 in Volume 2 of his *General Anatomy* (published in London), affirmed that 'one might think that nature has thus compensated the fair sex for their deficiency in many other parts' by giving women abundant hair. This fallacy persisted into this century, with the eleventh edition of the *Encyclopaedia*

Britannica firmly assuring its readers that male hair is naturally shorter than female hair among Western races. It was probably only the lack of examples to contradict this assertion that allowed it to persist. The 'sixties were to put paid to that, as today does the example of that admirable gardening guru, the well-named Bob Flowerdew, with his very long single plait.

Germaine Greer went on to observe that, while baldness is a sex-linked characteristic, it is not proper to maintain that women do not go bald. She observed that the intensity of sexual prejudice has resulted in the utter concealment of female baldness, which is much commoner than is generally supposed. Certainly the stereotype prevails. Hair hangs down over the body and implies modesty and with it femininity. Baldness of the head implies masculinity. Baldness elsewhere, by contrast, suggests femininity.

Whatever the perceptions, however, hair has the unique quality that it is, at the same time, both a part of us and separate from us. It has its own character. We can be its master or mistress, cutting it, colouring it, plaiting it, twisting it, shaving it and so on, yet it has the last laugh. This is because, when we die, it continues to grow upon our heads. If our coffins were to be reopened a year or so after death, we would be found becomingly covered with long tresses of hair (mortifyingly so in the case of a modern soldier particular about such things). Noel Coward once assured Eartha Kitt that not just on the head does hair continue to grow after death, but on the chest as well. Eartha Kitt protested that she had no hair on her chest, to which Noel responded: 'Oh, you women! You do give up so easily!'

In life as well as death, however, it seems that men could certainly equal women in the length of the hair on their heads. Indeed, they would more likely surpass them. *The Guinness Book of Records* tells of Swami Pandarasannadhi, whose hair, in 1949, was reported as being twenty-six feet in length. It also tells us that Ginny Bunford, the 'Birmingham Giantess' and the tallest woman in medical history, born in 1895, had her hair in two plaits down to her ankles. They were estimated at being eight feet in length, impressive yet somewhat insignificant in comparison to Swami Pandarasannadhi's twenty-six foot locks.

But it is hardly chivalrous to point out in this way that Bichat was so profoundly wrong. Let us instead turn to another Midland lass, Lady Godiva, who, with Venus and Eve, is surely the embodiment of long-haired femininity. Lady Godiva, however, stands apart from those two by drawing upon the practical aspect of long hair. Eve, when she became ashamed of her nakedness, clothed herself in leaves. Clearly she did not consider her hair sufficient cover to maintain modesty, whereas Lady Godiva, obliged by her husband to ride a horse naked through the streets of Coventry, put her hair to good use, modestly covering herself with it – not too modestly, however, to spoil a good picture (fig. 3). The townsfolk are said to have averted their eyes, but one feels sure they did quite the reverse and were fascinated to see the great lady's beautiful hair flowing so freely. The picture, dating from 1586, certainly gives viewers an opportunity to feast their eyes upon her.

Ted Polhemus maintains that hair has no practical use other than to make a personal, tribal or class statement

It also brings into the frame another aspect of female hair. A man with long hair is often described as 'leonine', a lion being masculine and likewise having a head of long hair (more so than a lioness). A long-haired woman is instead sometimes described as a 'filly', which the dictionary identifies either as a young female horse or a young woman, especially a lively one. Certainly, long hair and liveliness seem to go together, both in a mare and in a woman. This comparison of the human female with the equine surely has its base in the tossing mane that is common to both, unless cropped and (by implication) tamed. The similarity between the two is particularly evident in this picture, in which the long white tresses of the grey mare complement the long golden tresses of her rider.

Overlooking Lady Godiva's use of hair for modesty, Ted Polhemus maintains that hair has no practical use other than to make a personal, tribal or class statement, or so he says in Issue 19 of *Body Art*. Certainly groups, from guards officers to Hindu priests, use hair to help identify themselves. Desmond Morris, the animal behaviourist, concedes even less to the usefulness of human hair. In *Bodywatching* he sees it as being no more than a species identification mark. He writes:

> For more than a million years we were running around with almost naked bodies topped by a great mass of overgrown fur. While the hair on our trunks and limbs shrivelled to insignificance and exposed the whole of that skin surface to the open air, the hair on our scalps sprouted into a huge woolly bush or a long swishing cape. Unadorned and unstyled we must have looked amazing to other primates. What manner of ape was this?

Human, of course. However, running around with yards of hair sprouting from our heads is surely hardly justified if it is only there to differentiate us from the apes.

Hair also has an emotional function, not least in helping a woman to win her man. Rapunzel let down hers from the tower in which she was incarcerated, but not in an attempt to escape. On the contrary, she did so in order that her lover could climb up it to join her. The story, on the surface, is one of physical practicality (however fantastic). Underneath, it is one of raw sensuality.

It is that raw sensuality with which a long-haired woman can literally bind her man by winding her dark tresses round his neck. Dark because such a trap is sinister and such an ostensibly loving gesture could so easily lead to death. It is the concept of *la belle dame sans merci* capturing and perhaps destroying her knight at arms, 'lone and palely loitering'.

It is that sensuality, too, which leads a blonde to hold her long hair above her head and let it cascade down her back to where it brushes her buttocks. She does so for her own pleasure, before a mirror or beside

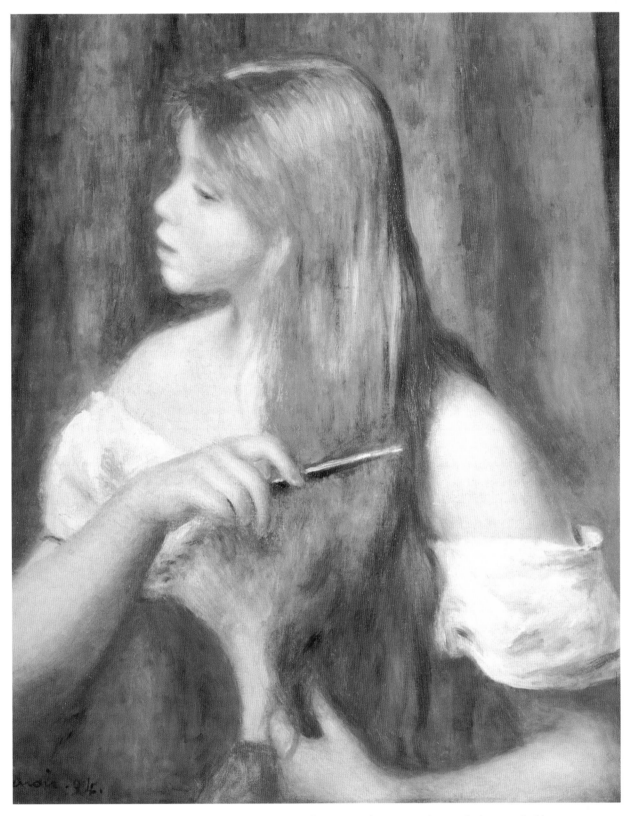

FIG. 4. Painful beauty — one can almost see this poor girl wince as she combs her tangled hair.
Pierre Auguste Renoir, *Blonde Girl Combing her Hair*, 1894 (Metropolitan Museum of Art, New York)

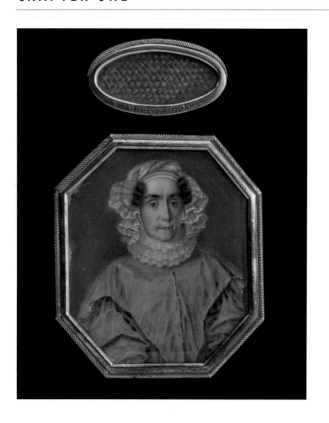

FIG. 5. The upper part of this double frame contains a lock of the hair of the lady depicted beneath it; this actual relic surely brings her closer to us than does her portrait.
Russian School, *Portrait of Praskovya Mikhailovna Tolstaya (1777–1844), with a latticed lock of her hair*, Russian School, nineteenth century
(Hermitage, St Petersburg)

a pool, but she surely hopes that a potential lover, known or unknown, will be watching. Blonde she may be, but not without guile. In the nineteenth century a woman with her hair down, let alone naked, was something a man could seldom hope to see, other than within the frame of a grand painting, in a brothel or as his own wife or mistress brushed her hair. The only exception would be the case of a child, such as the girl in fig. 4, whom Renoir has captured in a moment of absorption as she combs her hair, not easily but painfully, the comb tugging at her head. The picture demonstrates the impracticality of hair in its natural state; quite simply it gets tangled. The picture also evokes the strange paradox of hair being a part of one and yet separate. It is something that you have to hold out, because, unlike an arm or a leg, you have no physical way in which to move it otherwise than to toss it with your head.

Long hair presents a maintenance problem, worthwhile solving if you wish to maintain your lover's regard, but otherwise not unless you have a host of chambermaids. The nineteenth-century beauty the Empress Elizabeth of Bavaria certainly had plenty of these, but rather than have them bind up her hair she would defy convention and let it flow freely down the richest of ball gowns, not innocent and blonde like that of Renoir's girl, but sumptuously and seductively black and even more sumptuous than a child's. Endowed with great wealth and station, she was well endowed with the natural advantages of life too. Winner takes all.

A great lady may revel in the freedom of free-flowing hair, normally denied to all but the child. Children, however, may take pleasure in having their hair bound. Thoughtfully a child may suck the end of a plait, or feel its silky, rope-like texture and feel detached from and yet a part of it. There is something, too, about the ability to transform, to unplait that hair and hold it outstretched like the wings of an angel or an eagle. Then again it can be simply tied at the nape of the neck to create a swishing ponytail. It is all part of that fantasy born in small children who pretend to be ponies or mice, running around with tails tucked into the backs of their skirts or trousers. In this case, however, the tail is real. Or almost so, for it is, in truth, a mane.

Hair, then, has that capacity to assist fantasy and escape. It is a God-given trivial asset with which we can express ourselves in a way given to no other species, except perhaps for the horse swishing, the dog wagging or the cat twitching its tail.

Hair also conveys comfort when sleeping for those who unconsciously fondle their long hair, as a child might a teddy bear. As comforters, the hair and the breast go well together. The young baby reaches for both when first he comes to know his mother. Hair can also be used in an expression of defiance. Obviously we can tug at another's hair in anger, simulated or otherwise. But we can also bite or pull our own hair in a gesture partly of frustration and partly of what we would wish to inflict upon our adversaries if only we could get our hands and teeth upon them. Not for nothing is 'it makes one want to tear one's hair out' a time-honoured expression.

Fear, too, is conveyed by hair. The hackles of a dog do indeed stand on end. Literally he bristles. Human hair less visibly stands on end, but the hairs at the back of the neck tingle when we see a ghost. The dead hair comes to life as if in sympathy for the dead.

One way in which hair is unique is that it is a part of one's physical self that can be given to a lover or retained by grieving relatives after death. Setting aside the severed finger that a kidnapper might send to his hostage's family (or even the toenail or two that would have served the same purpose without causing permanent mutilation), as a personal memento only hair has that magical quality of being a pleasant and tangibly evocative reminder of its original owner. The portrait of Praskovya Mikhailovna Tolstaya (fig. 5) is doubtless faithful enough in itself, but it is the latticed lock of hair framed above it that brings the viewer close to the real person, rather than simply to an artist's attempt to capture her likeness.

We come finally from fantasy and extreme to something rather more mundane and yet universal. Leonardo da Vinci's *Mona Lisa* (fig. 6) is possibly the best-known painting of any woman ever painted. And yet she is not particularly beautiful, decorative or fashionable. This is a painting that is surely remarkable for the sitter, at least, being unremarkable. Just as there is little to distinguish her facially, so there is nothing exceptional about her hair. Parted in the middle, it simply frames her face. It does lead us forward, however, in our exploration of the fashion and fantasy of hair. So far we have been looking at women whose hair has been left naturally long, seldom or never cut so far as one can tell, whereas the *Mona Lisa* is a woman who has had her hair cut just below the shoulder, just like many millions of women today and in the past. The second point is that, were her head shaven, she would be seen as a distinctly different person. Even if inside herself she felt that she was just the same, to the outside world she simply would no longer be the *Mona Lisa*.

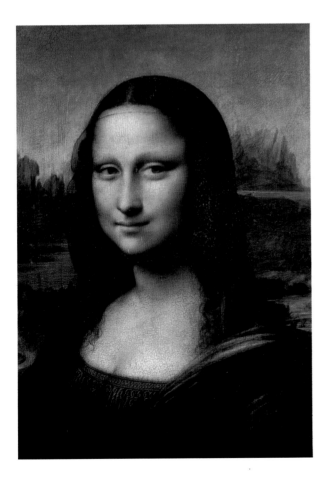

Fig. 6. Hair is as essential to a face as a frame is to a picture. Leonardo da Vinci, *Mona Lisa* (detail), c.1503–6 (Louvre Museum, Paris)

EGYPT

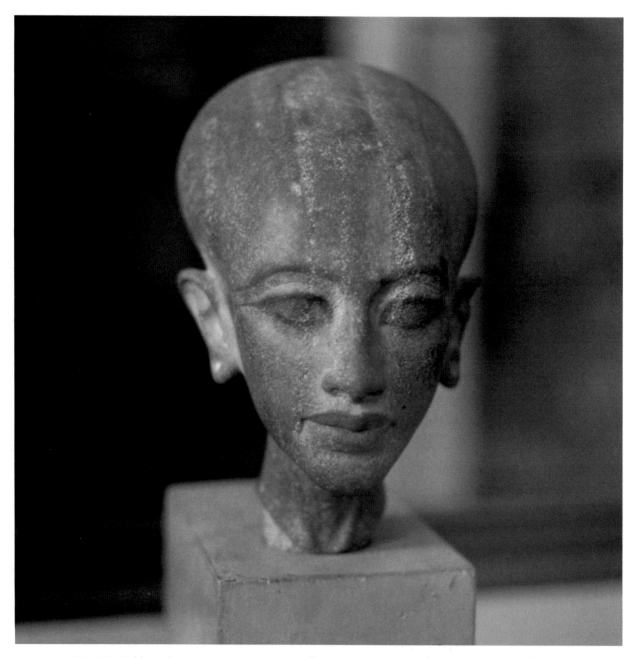

Fig. 7. Baldness has its beauty too – ironically, it was a reverence for the sacredness of hair
which dictated that this little princess should have her head shaved.
Portrait bust of a daughter of King Akhenaten, New Kingdom, c.1375 BC (Egyptian National Museum, Cairo)

Having pronounced that a hairless Mona Lisa would be unthinkable, the very next image we come to (fig. 7) is of a shaven-headed girl with remarkably similar eyebrows, eyes, nose and lips. This could indeed be a hairless Mona Lisa. Instead, she is Egyptian, the daughter of King Akhenaten, who lived in the fourteenth century BC, some two thousand seven hundred years before the Mona Lisa was painted. This little princess was shaven-headed for religious, social and climatic reasons. Indeed, almost universally in ancient Egypt, and certainly in royal and priestly circles, all heads, male and female, were shaved. When travelling abroad, however, the hair would be allowed to grow, not to conform with those being visited but to avoid the problem of disposing of hair trimmings in a strange land. Considered to be sacred and an integral part of the body, hair had to be carefully disposed of when shown. So it is, perversely, in a profound reverence for hair that our little princess has a shaven head. If hair could fall into evil hands, better by far that it should not be allowed to grow in the first place.

This is not to say that the Egyptians did not indulge in styling hair; quite the reverse. It was partly their delight in elaborate hairstyles that brought about the near-universality of the shaven head. In a hot climate, where a princess has an elaborate or abundant hairstyle, vermin can take a hold. This was especially the case when, again for religious reasons, the hair was seldom washed. The fear was that the guardian spirit of the head might be disturbed. In Persia, Herodotus reports that the king's head was washed only on his birthday, amid great ceremony. Herodotus also maintained that shaving the head from an early age toughened the skull. Similar thinking prevailed in Egypt. Right or wrong, it was certainly good for business, both for barbers and wig makers.

While our Egyptian princess is shown shaven-headed in fig. 7, another princess, in fig. 8, is seen wearing a wig. The surmounting headdress apart, this is the Mona Lisa with her hair restored to her, dark with a central parting, falling further below the shoulder maybe, but no further than the breast. Centuries and civilisations apart, one girl's hair natural and the other's artificial,

the two girls of a similar age surely have surprisingly much in common.

Typically, Egyptian wigs – the Hathor wig among them – were divided into three parts, one flowing down the centre of the back and one on each side reaching to the breasts. They must have been easy to put on, with the three sections guiding them into the proper position. Importantly, the ears were not covered, forming shell-like centres to the swirl of the wig around them. The wig usually had a brow band, like the brim of a cap, running around the head just above the ears. It was

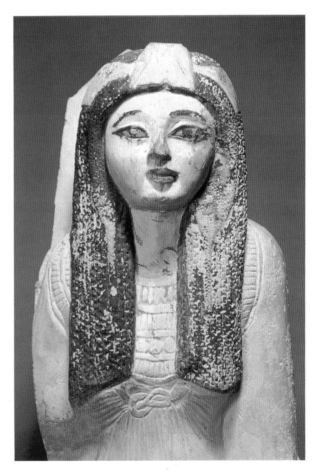

FIG. 8. This could be the girl in fig. 7 wearing a wig of human or horse hair. Both bear an uncanny similarity to the *Mona Lisa*, despite the centuries and civilisations which separate them.
Bust of an Egyptian princess

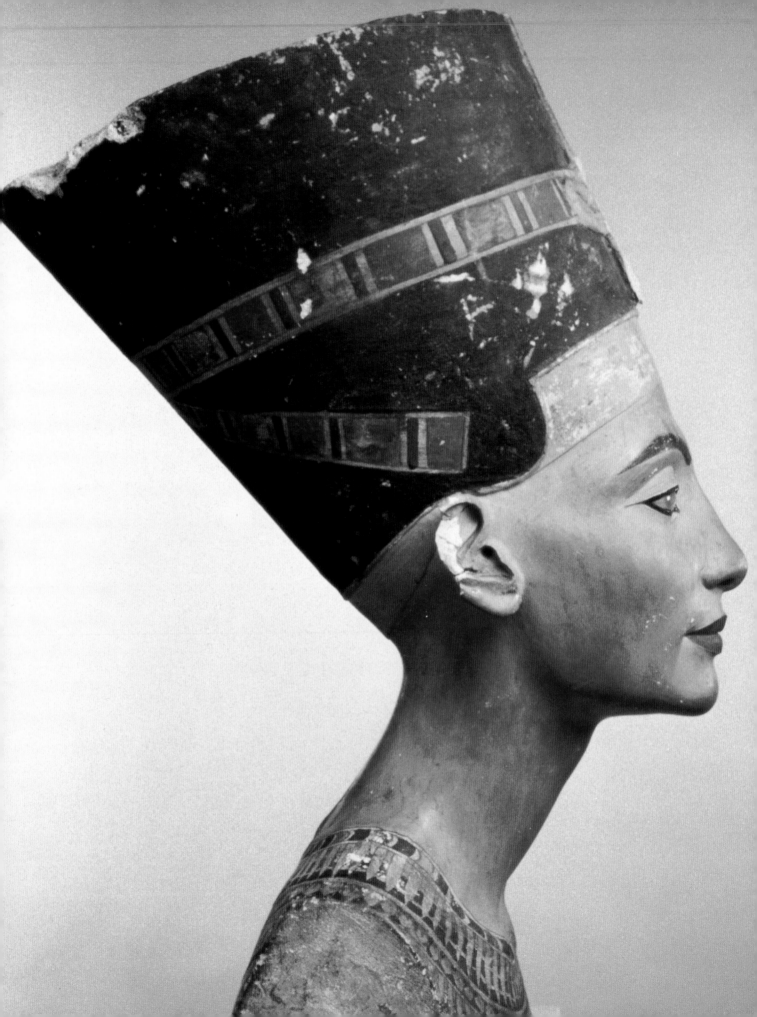

obviously an essential part of the wig's construction, but it also simulated a crown or a ribbon that one might wear to secure one's own hair, if one had any. While the wig itself was, in effect, a hat or crown and its length and style had some bearing upon the wearer's status, it could sometimes have a further embellishment such as the modius, which was rather like a little pillbox hat.

Sooner or later it was bound to seem easier for a woman not to wear a wig, but to place her headdress directly onto her bald head. The effect can be stunning, as evidenced by the bust of Queen Nefertiti (fig. 9). However, here there is a degree of artifice in the style of the headdress itself. Continuing the lines of the nape of her neck and her forehead, it almost suggests that she has long black hair raised high above her head and bound by a jewelled ribbon. The headdress clearly had the advantage over either a wig or natural hair of being much cooler and more easily maintaining its shape. Indeed, the wig as an alternative to one's own hair must surely have been of rather doubtful benefit. The best wigs were made of human hair, probably imported, but others were made of wool and palm-leaf fibres, even straw. While they were ventilated and could give some protection from the sun, they were sometimes uncomfortably warm indoors. This is said to have given rise to the custom of placing perfumed wax cakes on the wigs of visitors, the idea being that the melting wax would have a pleasantly cooling effect.

The use of wigs certainly provided more scope for flights of fancy than one might risk with one's own hair. Black was the favourite colour, but others – such as red, blue and green – were experimented with. And if one

Wigs were not always so formalised and artificial in appearance, however. They could even be intended to deceive one into thinking that the wearer had her own hair

was being less than natural in one's approach to one's wig, why not have a beard as well? This might seem rather strange for a queen, but, since beards were often of straw and hardly natural in appearance in any case, why should that be a hindrance? Another strange little addition would be the so-called 'lock of youth'. A child, when first shaven, would be allowed to retain just one lock of hair. The age-old desire to continue to look youthful led to that lock often being retained, hanging down from beneath the wig. Alternatively, a false representation of it would be attached to the wig.

Wigs were not always so formalised and artificial in appearance, however. They could even be intended to deceive one into thinking that the wearer had her own hair. Often they would indeed be made of natural hair, which was braided and the braid set in beeswax, not something one would relish if it were one's own hair. In the eighteenth dynasty some Thebans wore many-braided shoulder-length wigs. The braids would swing alluringly from their headbands, particularly when they were dancing. Rather more sedate are the man and his wife seen in fig. 10, also from Thebes and from the same dynasty. But they are not dancers. Indeed to our eyes they could be sitting in front of the fire, looking at something improving on television. Their less natural, rather more formal wigs indicate status: that of an official and his wife. The square cut of the woman's slightly longer wig and the rounded style of her husband's doubtless spoke volumes about their precise place in society. Who knows, too, whether she did not discard

FIG. 9. Queen Nefertiti wears a hair-like head-dress on her shaven head.
Bust of Queen Nefertiti, side view, from the studio of Thutmose at Tell el-Amarna, Egyptian, eighteenth dynasty, fourteenth century BC (Bode-Museum, Berlin)

her more formal wig for a lively braided number from time to time, all set to go 'clubbing'?

Such flippant comments would clearly never come from a serious Egyptologist. However, they do point to an important fact about Egyptian hairstyles, which is that although they come from a distant civilisation spanning more than three thousand years, they have had a profound influence on hairstyles ever since. There is something very up-to-date about them.

The little princess in fig. 7 could be the shaven-headed model of today. The ancient modius hat has an element of modern Parisian chic about it. Queen Nefertiti's headdress in fig. 9 would be at home in the *art deco* period of the twentieth century, either as a mascot on a long-bonneted motor car or as the carefully sculpted hair of a stylish society lady, cigarette-holder in hand. The dancing girls with their many little braids could come straight out of a nightclub of today. Echoing the concept of the 'lock of youth' surviving as an addition to a wig is the tiny bow found at the back of today's riding cap, the last vestige of the pigtail of the eighteenth-century postillion. Queen Nefertiti's high brow (brows cannot get higher than when your head is shaven) is likewise a precursor of the way in which an English queen, Queen Elizabeth I, plucked her forehead in order to be (literally) 'a highbrow'. Finally, the wigs worn by the couple in fig. 10 are remarkably like those still to be seen on the heads of English judges. Then, as now, wigs were symbols of status far removed from any attempt at faithfully replicating natural hair. It is not just Egypt's tombs but also her hairstyles that have been plundered down the ages. Their stylish artifice contrasts with the natural flowing character of hair left to its own devices, and that is surely the secret of their long-lasting and ever fresh fascination.

Queen Nefertiti's high brow (brows cannot get higher than when your head is shaven) is likewise a precursor of the way in which an English queen, Queen Elizabeth I, plucked her forehead in order to be (literally) 'a highbrow'

Fig. 10. The length and shape of the wigs worn by this husband and wife are symbols of status, just like those worn by some judges today and just as artificial. A man and his wife, Thebes, Egyptian, late eighteenth dynasty, c.1350 BC (British Museum)

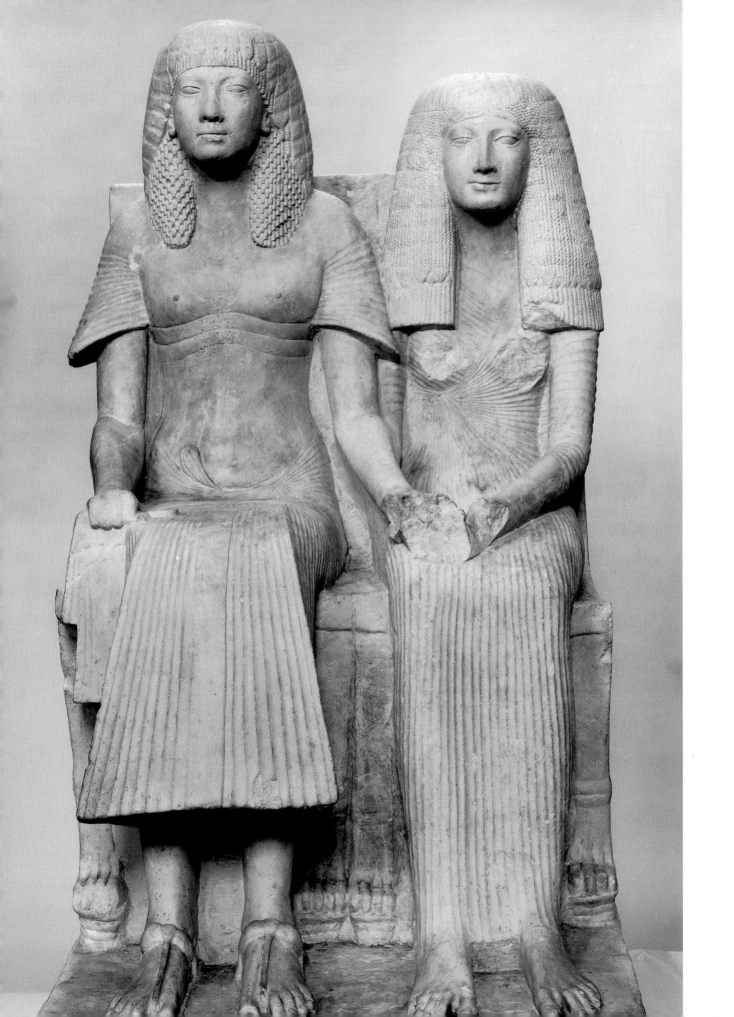

GREECE, ROME AND THE HOLY LAND

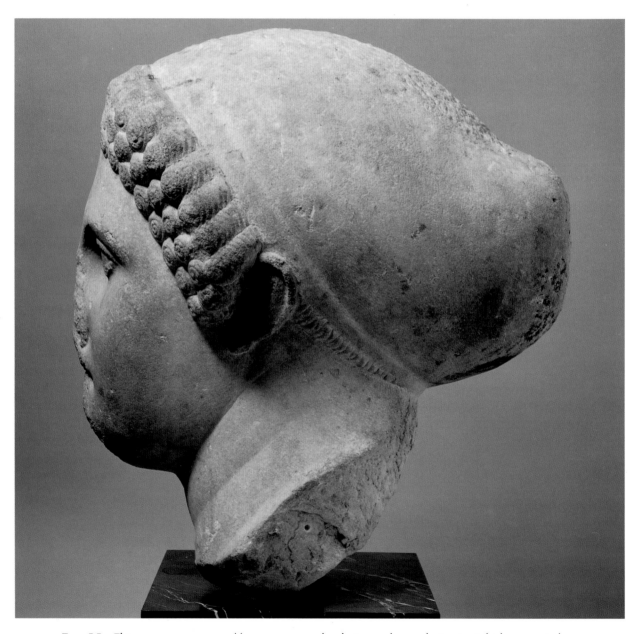

FIG. 11. This woman wears a *sakkos* or cap over her hair, much as a hairnet might be worn today. Bust of a woman from the mausoleum at Halikarnassos, c.350 BC (British Museum)

The image of shaven-headed Egyptians wearing voluminous wigs is, of course, contrary to the perception of Ancient Egypt promulgated by Elizabeth Taylor playing Cleopatra wearing her own luxuriant hair. That, however, was not just a Hollywood flight of fancy. Roman influence had indeed brought the fashion for wearing one's own hair into Egyptian society. In turn, the way in which that hair was worn had come from Greece to Rome. There were, in any event, similarities between the three civilisations, particularly when it came to the headdress. A Greek goddess would wear a high 'polos' or crown, bearing a superficial resemblance to an Egyptian goddess wearing her modius of a thousand years before. We have already likened the modius to the pillbox hat; the polos, in turn, reminds us of the hats that can be seen to this day on the heads of Greek Orthodox priests.

Still in the realms of headgear, the woman in fig. 11, with her hair parted from ear to ear and a row of tight curls arching over her forehead, has the rest of her hair secured within a cap called a 'sakkos'. The outline of the bun of hair at the back of her head is clearly visible through it. Here is headgear worn to control hair, rather than to cover a shaven head as so often would have been the case in Egypt. A further radical difference stems from the way in which Greek civilisation equated a low forehead with beauty, quite the reverse of the Egyptian view. Accordingly, the woman in her sakkos, with her front hair curled low across her brow and her back hair secured in a low cap to the nape of the neck, could not be more in contrast to Queen Nefertiti in fig. 9, with her high forehead and headgear rising up from the brow in the front and the nape of the neck at the back. It is not just a thousand years and a few hundred miles that separate these two, but an entirely different concept of beauty and fashion.

However, it is perhaps unfair to compare an Egyptian queen with a somewhat bourgeois Greek matron. Far more quintessentially Greek in terms of style and beauty must surely be the young woman in fig. 12. The bust of the woman in the sakkos dates from 350 BC, while this young woman comes from a slightly later period (325–275 BC). She has her hair secured with a broad band of material wound round her head and tied in a

Roman influence had brought the fashion for wearing one's own hair into Egyptian society

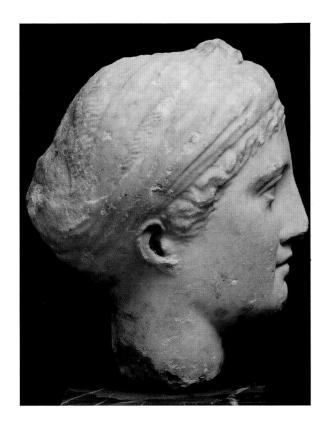

FIG. 12. A young woman with her hair secured by a hidden band of material wound round her head, low over her brow. In Greece a low forehead was an essential element in the classical pursuit of the beautiful. Greek woman, 325–275 BC

knot. The Egyptian wig might have hidden the hair, if there was any to hide, but here the band of material is itself hidden by the hair folded over it. The hair is secured in a bun at the back with a forelock tied in a knot at the front, bringing the hair both low over the forehead and low over the nape of the neck. Meanwhile the hair over the top of the head acts as a cap within what amounts to a wreath made from the girl's own hair. The use of a broad band of material around the head – a fillet – was a characteristic of the hairstyles of both men and women, deriving from the way a young male athlete would bind up his hair before running, a practice first adopted centuries before.

Another classic hairstyle was the 'lampadion'. The hair was drawn to the crown of the head and tightly

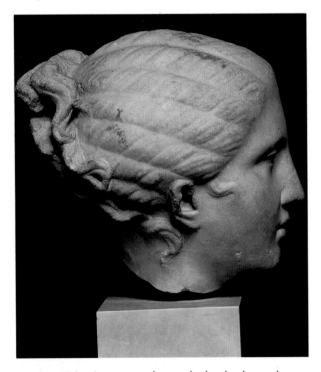

FIG. 13. One can understand why this hairstyle was known as the 'melon', with the hair drawn back in segments from the forehead and secured in a knot at the back.
Young Greek girl with a melon coiffure
(British Museum)

bound to look like a miniature version of a flaming beacon, hence the name. A further enduring Greek hairstyle dating from the fifth century was the so-called 'melon' modelled by the young girl in fig. 13. Her hair is drawn back in segments from the forehead and secured in a knot at the back. Between each of her many partings, and running the length of her head, the hair is separated and curled, arranged in parallel rows. An advantage of the style was that it could be adapted to either short or long hair, the effect from the front being just the same. If it was short, it would need to be secured with fillets; if it was long, the strands could be bound together in a twisted knot at the back.

It is impressive to see these hairstyles frozen, so to speak, in marble. But if they were challenging enough for the sculptor with his chisel, they must have been presented an even greater challenge to the hairdresser. A goddess, presumably, could call on supernatural aids to help her with her coiffure. Mere mortals would have to struggle long and hard to achieve the desired effect. The tools to do so were remarkably similar to those of today, though rather more elegant, as testify meticulously decorated ivory combs surviving from the period.

Elaborate examples of hairstyles from the later period of the Ancient Greek civilisation epitomise all that is elegant and beautiful. Earlier Greece, however, could be said to encapsulate the stylish and practical. A female athlete might have had her hair bound around a fillet at the front and plaited at the back, complementing the sensible above-the-knee hemline of her skirt. Such a girl would have been equally at home, perhaps, on a tennis court of the 1930s, just like the player of that time personified by John Betjeman's heroine, Joan Hunter-Dunn. In much the same way, a later and more elaborate Greek goddess could be mistaken for an eighteenth-century beauty. The one is an example of the functional, and the other of the beautiful, being handed down the centuries from Ancient Greece.

However it was worn, the Greeks were superstitious about the nature and quality of hair. Alexanna Speight, writing in *The Lock of Hair*, published in London in 1871, maintained that it was the custom for the Greeks:

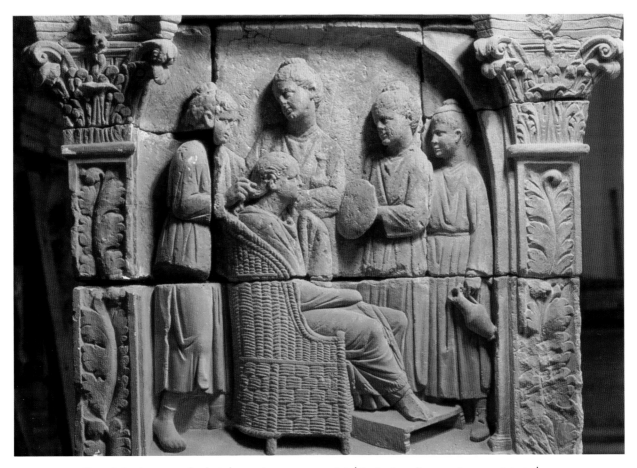

FIG. 14. A visit to the hairdresser's was as convivial in Ancient Roman times as it is today.
Stone bas relief of a hairdresser, Roman, c. second century AD (Rheinisches Landesmuseum, Trier)

… to hang the hair of the dead on their doors previous to interment, and the mourners not infrequently tore, cut off or shaved their own hair which they laid upon the corpse, or threw into the pile to be consumed along with the body of the relation or friend whose loss they lamented.

Care was sometimes taken, likewise, only to cut the hair at the time of the new moon. It would make hairdressing salons periodically crowded and otherwise empty if the same practice were to be followed today.

Imitation is said to be the sincerest form of flattery, and the Romans were certainly very sincere in the way they adopted Greek hairstyles. It was fashionable to own Greek slaves and sculpture. A slave would have his head shaved and, understandably, grow back his hair on obtaining his freedom. More usefully, a slave girl could have her hair cut from time to time to augment the coiffure of her Roman mistress. A copy of a Greek statue would often stand in a Roman villa. The lady of the house might copy the hairstyle it depicted, using a lock or two of Greek slave-girl hair to make good any deficiencies of her own.

So it is that we see sculpture not just as a work of art or a record of a particular individual, but as something that influenced fashion in hairstyles, from land to land and from age to age. Today, in order to select a style, one might flip through the pages of *Vogue* or *Cosmopolitan*. In the past one would have taken a stroll through the sculpture gallery – and sculpture, though hardly as practical and easily circulated as the modern magazine, does have the compensating qualities of

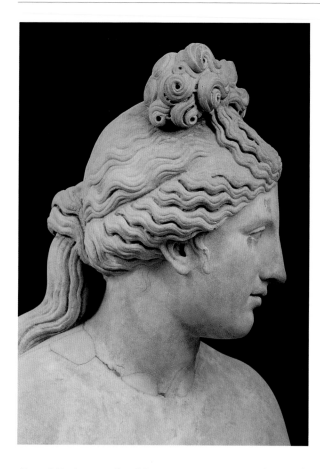

FIG. 15. Livia, wife of Emperor Augustus, set the trend for wearing a nodus or knot over the brow of the head. Empress Livia, wife of Augustus, 25–1 BC, Roman

durability and of being three-dimensional. You can walk around a sculpture and see what the hairstyle looks like from the back. It has to be said, however, that the sculptor might not always be too concerned to show you how the hair, in reality, would have been secured. In the same way a hairdresser of today might secure some elaborate hair style by spraying it with fixative, to hold it just long enough for a photograph to be taken, without any concern for its maintenance in a real-life situation.

Sometimes, indeed, in the spirit of Roman practicality and innovation, sculptors would make the hair on a portrait bust detachable. Accordingly, a beautifully sculpted marble coiffure could be removed and replaced

with one of a later fashion. One wonders if some hairdressers did not have such visual aids readily to hand to demonstrate the various options open to their customers, a precursor of yesterday's identikit and today's computer simulation.

The Romans, of course, created their own hairstyles and scrutinised the effect with care, as in the case of the pampered customer seen in fig. 14 visiting a Roman hairdresser's. One attendant holds a mirror, another a pitcher of water, while a third attends to the back hair. The fourth is presumably the salon proprietor, encouraging her minions and engaging the customer in reasonably untaxing and suitably flattering conversation. Little changes over the years.

A hairdresser's establishment was frequented by the middle classes, the upper classes having their hair dressed by their slaves. Whether at home or in the salon, however, the hair could well be distinctly oily, since many people considered it unlucky to wash their hair more than once a year, in a superstition thereby persisting down the centuries.

Roman men, generally speaking, wore their hair short, combed forward and curled, sometimes artificially so. It was a style that was to influence later female hair-styles with which the name of Titus (AD 40?–81), the son of Emperor Vespasian, was most frequently associated.

In her own time Livia (fig. 15), the wife of Emperor Augustus, popularised a nodus or knot over the brow of the head. The remaining hair was drawn back on either side and tied likewise at the back. This very personal style was closely copied between 25 and 1 BC. An example can be seen in fig. 16, which shows a husband flanked by his wife and daughter. His wife (to the right) has the distinctive nodus, but his daughter (to the left) has moved on to the simple, centre-parted fashion, which indeed the empress later adopted. In fact, this simpler style harked back to classical Greece. This was the style that Cleopatra adopted, the style thus going from Greece to Egypt via Rome.

Roman ladies, however, were not necessarily known for their restraint. From the first century AD comes an example of elaborately built-up front hair with ringlets hanging to either side (fig. 17). Probably only the curls on the brow are her own, but it is the hair above the brow that forms the principal feature of the so-called orbis style. This arc of hair ranging from ear to ear was, initially, self-supporting. However, in its later manifestations it was clearly aided by a metal frame resting on the ears.

Juvenal gives a splendid account of an orbis being set up:

> So high they pile her head, such tiers on tiers
> With weary hands they pile, that she appears
> Andromandroche before – and what behind?
> A dwarf, a creature of another kind.

These words reflect how the hairstyle was indeed one that was all front and no back.

The Egyptians copied the Greeks via the Romans in returning to a fashion for wearing one's own hair. In return they reminded the Romans of the convenience of the wig, espoused by them for so many centuries before. A Roman example of a woman wearing a wig is shown in fig. 18. Here the natural hair is seen clearly at the front of the head and the wig is worn like a cap, curling round the ears. The woman's back hair, in a plait, peeps out from beneath the wig. It is almost as if she has flung the wig on to go shopping, having despaired of her own hair when catching sight of it in the hall mirror. However, since this is not a snapshot but a marble portrait for which the subject deliberately posed, she is probably rather showing off her latest 'fashion accessory'. It certainly gives her a degree of flexibility. She can let down her own hair and have it long and flowing, or wear it in combination with the wig's shorter style. Wigs (blonde ones made of hair from Germany) were also worn with rather less propriety by prostitutes, who were required to identify themselves in this way. However, the situation changed when the blonde hair became fashionable within society. Roman ladies would seek to bleach their hair or, like the prostitutes before them, wear blonde wigs made from the shorn locks of Germany maidens.

Concurrent with the Egyptian dynasties and the rise

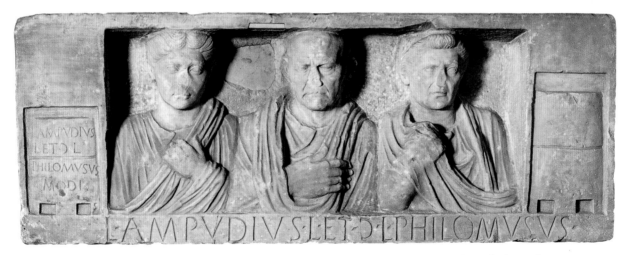

FIG. 16. In this family group, the man has the short 'senatorial' hairstyle; to the right his wife copies the Empress Livia with her nodus, while to the left his daughter has the more classical central parting to which, by then, the Empress herself had probably reverted. Luceus Ampudius Philomus with his wife and daughter, marble relief, 15–5 BC, Roman

and fall of the Greek and then the Roman civilisations were the times and customs of those who lived in the Holy Land throughout the events of the Old and New Testaments. One would expect their heritage to be

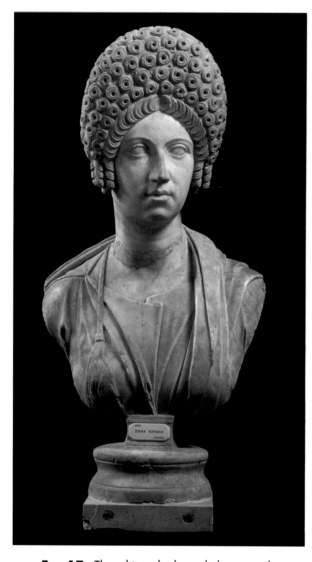

FIG. 17. The orbis style depended upon curls being built up over a metal frame and further curls being added, often shed by slaves for the purpose.
Marble portrait bust of a lady, AD c.69–96, Roman, Flavian dynasty
(Museo Archeologico Nazionale, Naples)

equally rich and influential, and so it might have been were it not for the Jewish commandment that there be no graven images. Accordingly there is little illustrative material to assist comparison and imitation.

It is tempting to turn to the paintings of the nineteenth-century pre-Raphaelites that depict biblical scenes in a highly realistic style, showing male and female subjects with the long robes and long hair widely assumed to typify that period. But perhaps the only information that we can reliably turn to is the exhortation in Leviticus 9:27 to men that: 'Ye shall not round the corners of your heads, neither shalt thou mar the corners of thy beard.' Women, after marriage, were obliged to keep their hair covered. In short, there are no pictures and, even if there were, there would be little to be seen of mature female hairstyles, if keeping your hair under a veil can be so described.

During this period, however, there are certainly records of hairstyles specific to other races and tribes, illustrating the use of hairstyles to identify groups, which Ted Polhemus sees as hair's main function (as opposed to Desmond Morris's more basic concept of hair simply identifying the human species). So it was that Hittite man would have a plaited braid hanging from just forward of his ear and, by contrast, a shaven patch above it. A Moabite would have his hair long at the back, but shaven to a line running from ear to ear at the front. However, such idiosyncrasies were to have little lasting implication for hairstyles down the ages. They may be evoked today in the hairstyle of some young man trying to shock his parents, but it is hardly likely that he would look to historical precedent for justification.

The popular image of Christ having hair to just below the shoulder is, in fact, a reasonable one. This is the way in which one would assume that, unconstrained by fashion, most men would have worn their hair. It would simply need to be no longer or shorter than would be convenient for working in a carpenter's shop or fishing on the Sea of Galilee. Likewise one would expect women to have worn their hair longer than many do today – long hair in the home being no constraint to practicality, particularly when worn under a veil. Furthermore, women working as spinners and weavers (literally 'the distaff side') would, because of their manual skills, be far more adept at plaiting their hair, and thus controlling it, than would a man. Alternatively, the married woman, keeping her head covered, might decide to sell her hair for export to assist in making all those wigs in Egypt or in Rome.

St Paul said that long hair was shame to a man but glory to a woman. However, he was speaking, initially at least, as an employee of the Roman Empire, anxious to copy the styles of the ruling race. In the well-known Old Testament story of Samson and Delilah, Samson derived his strength from his long hair, which Delilah then cut off, rendering him weak. Is this an allegory for the battle of the sexes with hair as the trophy to be won?

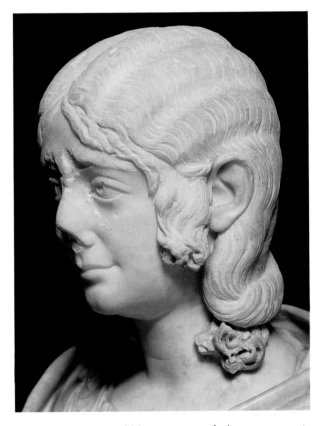

FIG. 18. A wig could be worn as a 'fashion accessory' with one's own hair clearly visible to the front and back, as here.
Marble portrait bust of a woman,
AD c.210–230, Roman

Most famous of all – she who atones for all protistution – must surely by Mary Magdalene, who anointed Christ's feet using her hair

In New Testament times, while St Paul might have considered hair to be a woman's glory, he was equally concerned that it should be covered, at least when at prayer, so as not to distract. Hair, free-flowing, would be the sign of a virgin and, covered, that of a married woman. The exception would be the hair of a prostitute. Most famous of all – she who atones for all prostitution – must surely be Mary Magdalene, who anointed Christ's feet using her hair. This must rank as one of the most sensual acts of obeisance imaginable. Fourteen hundred years later her hair was to be venerated in a painted panel in which the unknown 'Master of the St Mary Magdalen' showed his saint wearing her hair as if it were a long cloak, something practical and modest, rather than sensual and flagrant. Later, in the seventeenth century, she was to be depicted again with long tresses but somewhat unnecessarily (surely) with a bare bosom. These are images not of our time, nor yet of hers. They only serve to highlight that the principal fact we know about her is that she had long, uncovered hair, rather shocking in someone not a virgin but wonderful in the way she used it to anoint the feet of Christ.

So, however brilliantly illustrated our children's bibles may be, we can gain only a hazy picture of how hair was actually worn during this era in the Holy Land. We see men wearing long hair in defiance of the styles of their rulers, girls whose flowing hair was a symbol of virginity, or temptation, and married women with their heads decently covered. However, despite such scant information, one somehow detects a notion of purity and simplicity which would influence styles in generations to come, particularly in societies driven by Christian belief.

FROM THE MEDIEVAL TO THE RENAISSANCE

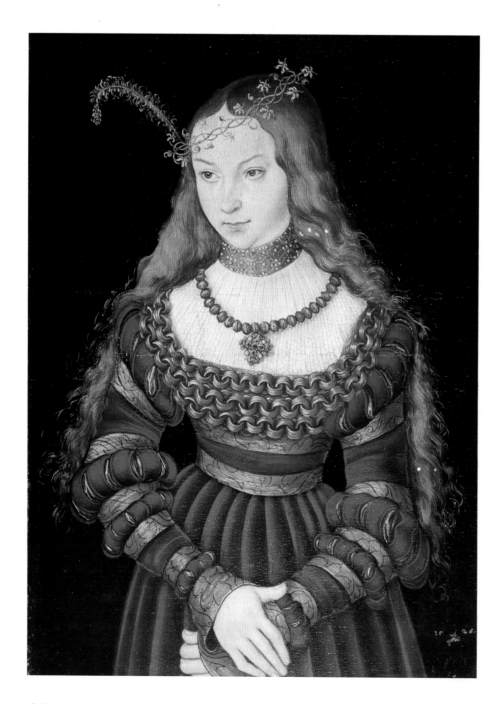

FIG. 19. A real princess with the long flowing hair of a bride.

Lucas Cranach the elder (1472–1553), *Princess Sybille of Cleves as a Bride* (Schlüssmuseum, Weimar)

Just as it is tempting to illustrate hairstyles from biblical times with splendid pre-Raphaelite paintings by nineteenth-century artists such as Holman Hunt, so it would also be tempting to illustrate the hairstyles of the Dark Ages – Arthurian knights and maidens, shown in a golden glow with flowing, unrestrained locks – by using examples from the same imaginative school. It is hardly less authentic, however, to illustrate the Dark Ages with a picture from the late fifteenth century (fig. 19), over a thousand years on

> However, from whatever period except our own, a princess has long, flowing hair— or so any little girl would have told you in the days before Diana

from the Roman girl with her wig in fig. 10. But then the Dark Ages would not be the Dark Ages had we illustrated records from them.

However, from whatever period except our own, a princess has long, flowing hair – or so any little girl would have told you in the days before Diana. Fig. 19 shows a princess who must surely be the personification of this concept. This is not a fictional representation but a contemporary picture of a real person. Princess Sybille of Cleves, painted by Cranach as a bride, has her hair flowing over her shoulders and down past her waist. Its golden red colour is echoed in the colour of her dress. Her breast, discreetly covered in lace, is outlined on the bust by material bound in such a way as to simulate plaits of the same colour as her hair. Another feature of the picture is one that we are accustomed to even in the press photographs of today; it is that a photograph or painting of a person usually stretches down as far as the ends of their hair. If the hair is short we seldom see below the neck, but the photographer or, in this case,

the artist can never resist showing the full extent of the hair. One's eye is therefore drawn down the hair, taking in with it the figure and the clothes (as here) or lack of them (as in Botticelli's Venus of the same period).

No race is identified by red hair. It is an individual anomaly, often associated with freckles. This Cranach beauty stands perhaps as a figurehead, representing all redheads, taunted, doubtless as much out of envy as fear, with names such as 'Carrot-top' or 'Hothead'. To those who have so suffered, she is surely a splendid vindication of this oft ridiculed (or secretly envied) colour.

There is a poignancy, too, in the moment in which Cranach has captured this little princess. It is the day of her marriage and, from now on, her hair will be largely hidden from view under a matronly veil.

From natural redheads we turn to unnatural blondes. During this era, the ladies of Venice had a passion for bleaching their hair. So dedicated were they in their pursuit of fair hair that special verandas and turrets sprouted from the tops of Venetian palaces and houses. Here they would sit in the sun, sometimes wearing a broad-brimmed hat without a crown, through which they would draw their hair and spread it out, so as to bleach it. In 1589 Cesare Vecellio reported that

> the houses in Venice are commonly crowned with little constructions in wood, resembling a turret without a roof. On the ground these lodges or boxes are formed of masonry, floored like what are called terrazzi at Florence and Naples.

He goes on to tell us that

> it is in these that the Venetian women may be seen as often and indeed oftener, than in their chambers. It is there that, with their head exposed to the full ardour of the sun during whole days, they strain every nerve to augment their charms.

Later, he tells us that:

> … during the hours that the sun darts its most vertical

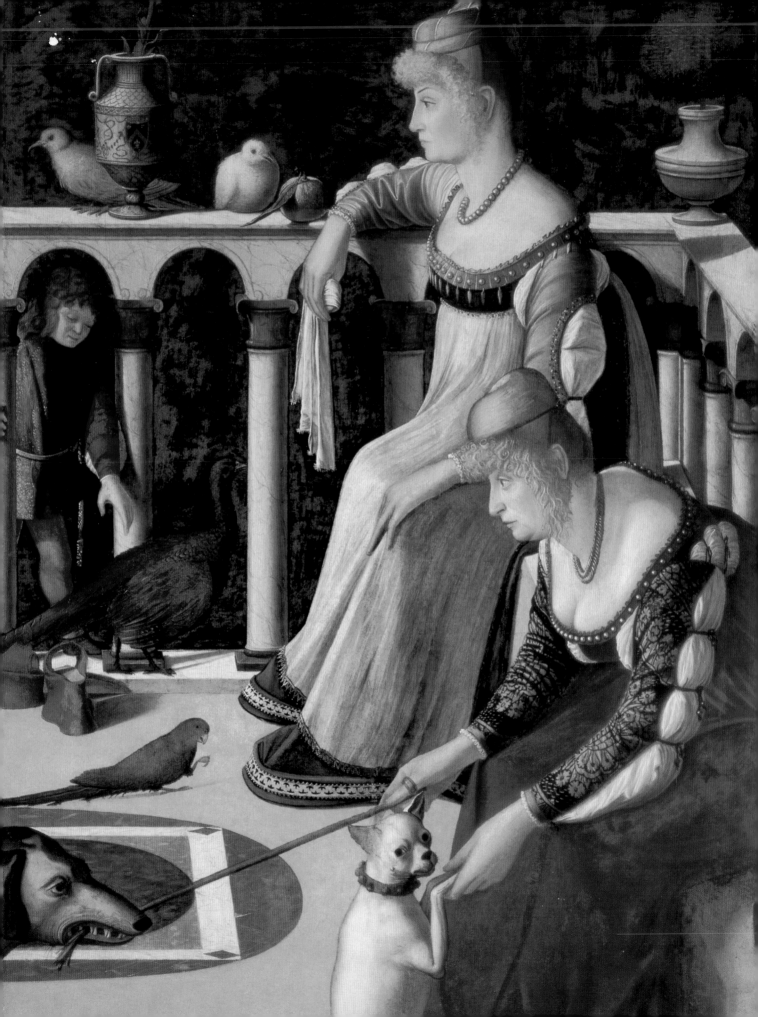

Local variations in traditional headgear, if no longer worn for everyday wear, are jealously guarded to this day throughout the Low Countries

and scorching rays, they repair to these boxes and condemn themselves to broil in them unattended. Sated there they keep on wetting their hair with a sponge dipped in some elixir of youth, prepared with their own hands or purchased. They moisten their hair afresh as fast as it is dried by the sun, and it is by unceasing renewal of this operation that they become what you see them – blondes.

Just such a pair of blondes can be seen in fig. 20. Their hair is up, rather than spread out in the sun, but it is piled high on top of their hatless heads. One holds a cloth as if to damp her hair. They certainly seem to be taking the beauty treatment very seriously. A feature of their coiffure, very up-to-date for the middle of the fifteenth century, is the way in which it is fluffed out and frizzed, a contemporary observing that 'the heare of woman that is laid over her forehead were called rolles'.

Moving North from Venice to the Netherlands one

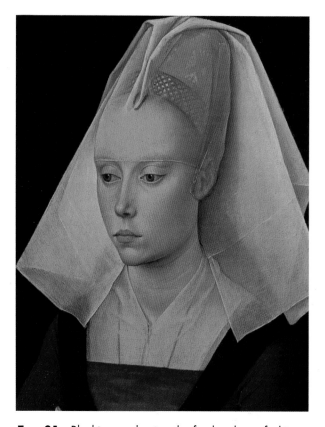

FIG. 21. Plucking or shaving the forehead was fashionable from the fourteenth century onwards, as clearly seen here under the girl's fine veil, passed over her headdress and secured beneath her ears. Workshop of Rogier van der Weyden, *Portrait of a Lady*, c.1450–60 (National Gallery, London)

FIG. 20. Giving nature a helping hand – Venetian ladies would sit bare-headed for hours in the sun hoping to bleach their hair, which they wore fluffed out and frizzed over the forehead in 'rolles'. Vittore Carpaccio, *Two Venetian Ladies*, fifteenth/sixteenth century (Civico Museo Correr, Venice)

comes to different customs. Hair would be contained within a 'mentonnière', contrived to look like horns. One finds just such a headdress in the famous painting of the 'Arnolfini marriage' (Portrait of Giovanni[?] Arnolfini and his Wife, National Gallery, London) and it was clearly a popular adornment in the artist Jan van Eyck's native Netherlands, around Maastricht. Local variations in traditional headgear, if no longer worn for everyday wear, are jealously guarded to this day throughout the Low Countries.

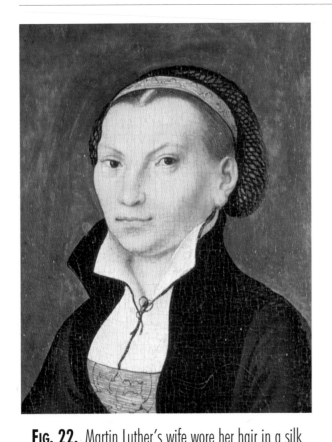

FIG. 22. Martin Luther's wife wore her hair in a silk bag inside a net.
Lucas Cranach the elder, *Katharina von Bora,*
future wife of Martin Luther, 1526
(Sammlungen auf der Wartburg, Eisenach)

to capture Katharina von Bora wearing another headdress (fig. 22). Her own hair is clearly visible, centrally parted, leading back to a brow band with a hairnet behind it, or so it would seem. In fact, the net is placed over silk, which matches the brow band. Her hair is bagged, unseen within. This lady was to become the wife of Martin Luther and fig. 23 is said to depict their daughter, Magdalena. Here a headband is again in evidence, but this time with no bag. The child's hair is left to flow unconstrained over both shoulders, very fine and very

At the same time that Cranach was painting in Germany, Leonardo da Vinci was exploring female beauty and, with it, fashion

blonde, enough to make a Venetian lady extremely jealous and possibly make an offer for it. Indeed, it is arranged in tresses almost as if ready for the hair dealer's scissors. More likely, though, it is ready for the hands of Katharina Luther to plait it, ready for school. That is as familiar a little chore in the households of long-haired girls today as it was then.

At the same time that Cranach was painting in Germany, Leonardo da Vinci was exploring female beauty and, with it, fashion. His portrait of Cecilia Gallerani (fig. 24) combines the two in ample measure. Here again is the band encircling the head like a diadem. Fascinatingly, the hair also appears to form a circle around the sitter's face, broken only by her central parting. Indeed, it seems to form a kind of chinstrap or mentonnière. Tantalisingly, the girl's head is turned in profile, so we cannot see how her hair is secured on the other side. However, it is likely that it sweeps down over her right ear, under the chin, then up over

Also from the Netherlands comes the lady in fig. 21, which illustrates the fashion from the fourteenth century onwards for women to pluck or shave their foreheads to move the hairline upwards. This Flemish lady also appears to be shaved to just above the ears while the eye is drawn still further upwards by the manner in which her hair is encased by a Flemish version of the polos favoured by her classical Greek counterpart. The whole is topped by a veil of finest silk coming down to her eyebrows and secured under the ear. She also echoes Queen Nefertiti and Egyptian fashion, though surely unconsciously so.

Later in the same century, in Germany, Cranach was

her left ear, to be folded with the hair on the left side of her parting. Then it comes across the top of her head at the point where we see the central parting concluding, finally to be finished in a tress (it does not appear to be braided) hanging down her back, secured by jewelled clasps, spaced at about four inches.

This transformation of long hair into a close-fitting skullcap, almost like the rubber swimming cap of today, is, it would seem, achieved by confining it in a very fine transparent veil. This has a gold embroidered brow band that follows the line of the eyebrows downwards, until it is hidden in the hair at the sides of the face. The result is to present the woman's face precisely as if it were a mask, disembodied from both her neck and the rest of her head by the dark framework of her hair. Our attention is focused on her face in precisely the same way that it would be focused upon that of a nun, except that the covering here is not a veil but the woman's own hair.

More open to the elements is the hair of the girl in the painting attributed to Domenico Ghirlandaio (fig. 25). She has a central parting with her hair pulled back behind her ears. It is constrained by a double hairband, looping first upwards to the crown of her head and then downwards around the bun at the back. It would seem that there is a further turn between the two, secured with a knot hidden behind a brooch just above her ear. But that is not all, because, enchantingly, the lower hair has been brought out from under the upper. These lower tresses on either side of the face, between the ear and the cheek, have had the attention of the curling tongs, while, by contrast, those behind have not. However, the greatest contrast is that this part of her hair, allowed to hang down, has been cut just above the shoulder, whereas the upper hair presumably, if unconstrained, would fall to the waist. It is an unusual but not impractical arrangement, the shorter hair framing the face and the longer hair, drawn back behind the ears, falling down the back, or put up (as here) in a bun. In terms of dressing long hair, this was certainly the age of inventiveness – at least in Italy, where the Renaissance arrived a century ahead of the rest of Europe.

This Italian inventiveness is further illustrated by fig. 26. Here, Alessandro Araldi shows his sitter, Barbara Pallavicino, in less-than-flattering profile, but helpfully so since the picture faithfully reproduces her headgear, front and back. The circlet that crowns her head, studded with gemstones, holds down the hair which, beneath it, swoops naturally from a central parting, down over the ears, to the nape of the neck. The singular aspect of this hairstyle, which was very fashionable at the time, is that the circlet also secures a skullcap to contain the hair at the back. The skullcap is worn almost vertically on the back of the head, and would therefore fall off were it not for the circlet. It is no ordinary skullcap,

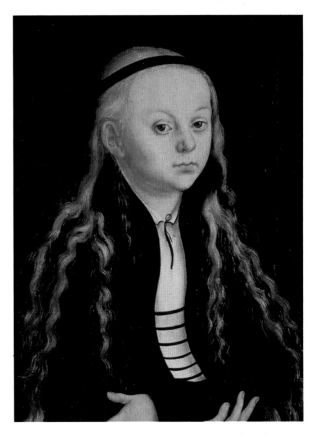

FIG. 23. The Luthers' daughter wore her hair loose beneath a headband.
Lucas Cranach the elder, *Portrait of a Young Girl*, possibly Magdalena Luther, daughter of Martin (Louvre Museum, Paris/Peter Willi)

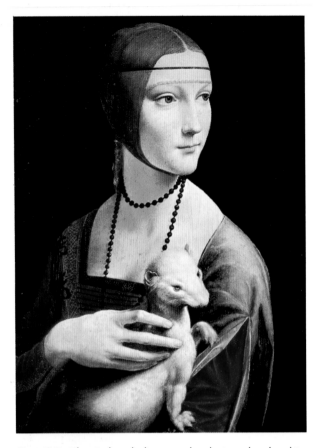

FIG. 24. This Italian lady wears her hair under the chin like today's rubber swimming cap or a contemporary nun's veil.
Leonardo da Vinci (1452–1519), *The Lady with the Ermine* (Cecilia Gallerani) (Czartorisky Musem, Krakow)

since her hair could be threaded more easily through the netting than my wife's could through the knitwear. Perhaps it is time that someone else made an attempt to revitalise this fascinating style, or a variation of it.

As it is, if the hairstyles of fifteenth-century Italy live on today, it is the male hairstyle which is most in favour, but adopted more by women than by men. Quite why can be addressed at the appropriate time, but it is perhaps not inappropriate that the example chosen here is a bust of Machiavelli, the great schemer (fig. 27). Machiavelli's hair is cut elliptically around the head, then brushed downwards from the crown and curled inwards. He looks much as a Roman emperor might have done had he forgotten to have his hair cut for five or six months. Equally emulated in later centuries was the haircut of the pageboy, which is all of one length and cut at the shoulder. Practical, yes; intriguingly androgynous on boys as yet unbearded, yes again. However, a further element of practicality comes into play when considering this style. Just as a maid might lose her hair to her mistress, so might a page. Marguerite de Valois usually had blond pages, not because she particularly liked having golden-headed boys about her, but rather because they could be shorn to provide blond hair for her wigs. One can just imagine the embarrassment of the page growing hair for his mistress, well below the shoulder, and the relief when she harvested her crop of hair from him.

Not surprisingly, women today do not look further back in history to emulate the hairstyles of William the Conqueror, said to have followed the Gallic fashion of shaving the back of the head, or Henry V (fig. 28) who

because it extends into an open lacework sausage, or funnel, into which the hair is trained from the nape of the neck downwards, towards her waist. The final embellishment is the large brooch with its large pendant which is pinned into the hair to hold the skullcap just above the ear. While this type of cap, with an extension for the hair, was fashionable in Italy at the time, it was certainly not so fashionable in England in the 1980s, when I had a knitted version of the headdress made for my wife. It has to be said that it was soon abandoned, because it was very difficult to stuff her hair into it. Doubtless, this lady found matters less complicated,

FIG. 25. Deceptively simple and charming, this girl's hairstyle is a complex mixture of the long, the short, the up, the down, the frizzed and the straight.
Attributed to Domenico Ghirlandaio, *Portrait of a Girl,* c.1490 (National Gallery, London)

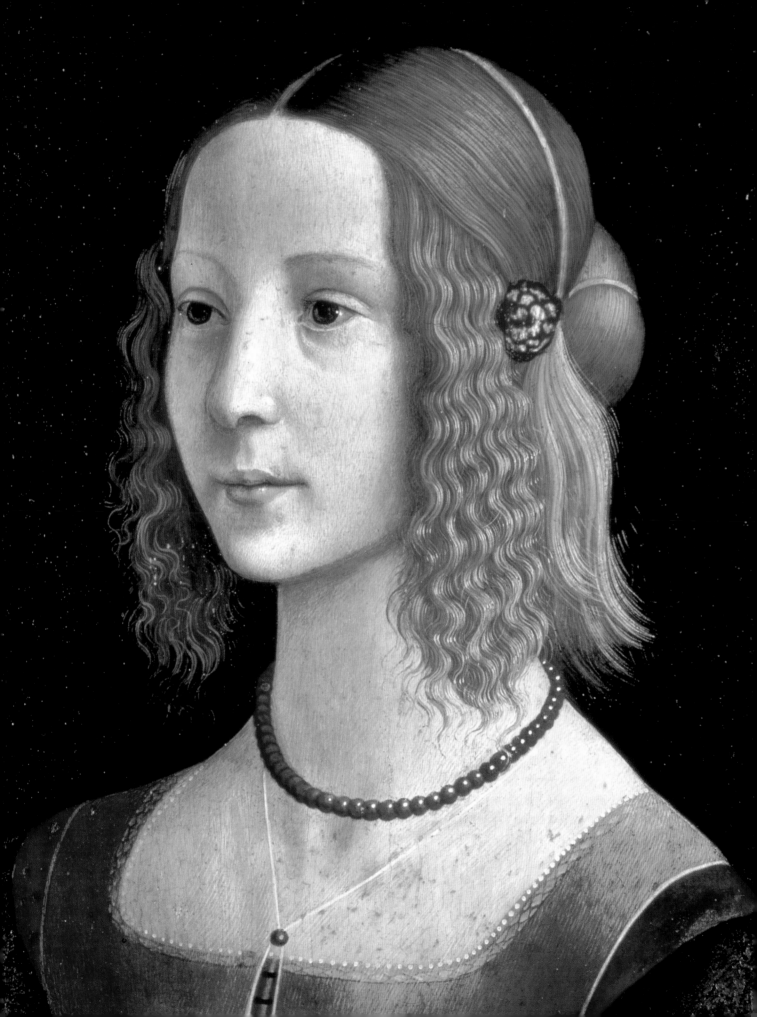

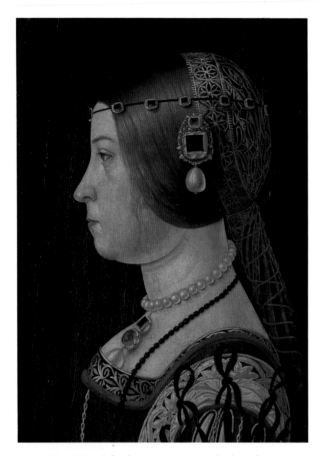

FIG. 26. A further variation on the hair-bag. Alessandro Araldi, *Portrait of Barbara Pallavicino*, c.1520–28 (Galleria degli Uffizi, Florence)

It is no ordinary skullcap, because it extends into an open lacework sausage, or funnel, into which the hair is trained on the nape of the neck downwards, towards her waist

of the head not been shaved. Whatever the reason, it is distinctly strange, as you will see if you visit Madame Tussaud's.

It is a relief to return from this diversion to the exquisitely female and the ever-inventive young ladies of sixteenth-century Italy with, in fig. 29, another

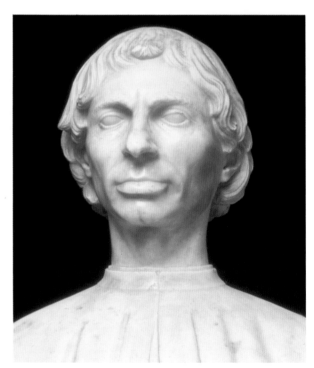

FIG. 27. The adult male hairstyle of the fifteenth century would be copied by women (and men) in the twentieth. Attributed to Antonio Pollaiolo (1433–98), marble bust of Niccolo Machiavelli (Bargello, Florence)

had his head shaved up to a line about two inches above his ear. The latter left a convenient cap of hair, doubtless to cushion his crown or helmet, but what reason William could have had for the fashion he adopted is hard to understand. It is almost as if the barber, enjoying a private joke, had carefully omitted to hold up the mirror to show him the back of his head before asking if there was anything he needed 'for the weekend'. One justification one might think of for this strange arrangement was to try to balance the nakedness of the front of the head with that of the back so as, from a distance, to confuse one's enemies. Again, it could have something to do with the fact that his helmet would have had chain mail hanging down behind it, in which hair could easily have become entangled had the back

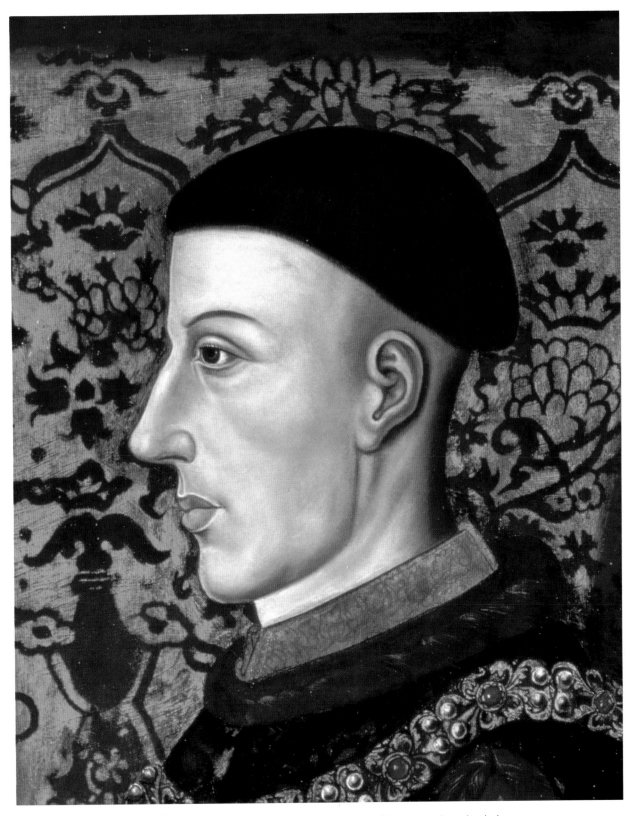

Fɪɢ. 28. Henry V had his head shaved leaving just a cap of hair to cushion his helmet or crown.
English School, Henry V (1387–1422), fifteenth century (National Portrait Gallery, London)

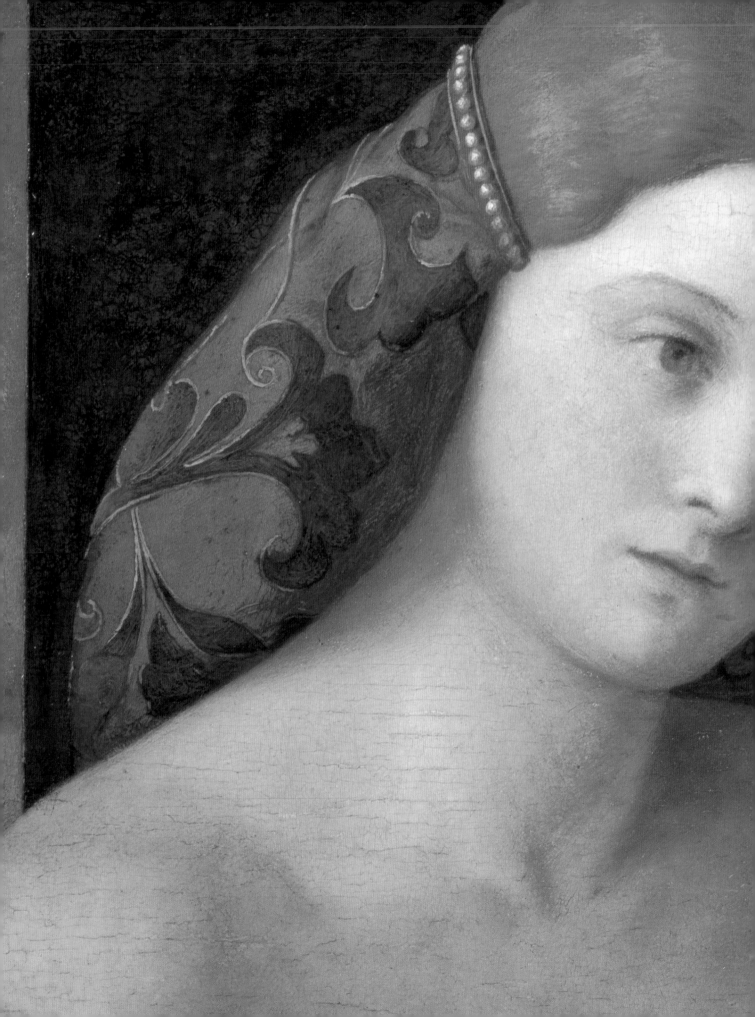

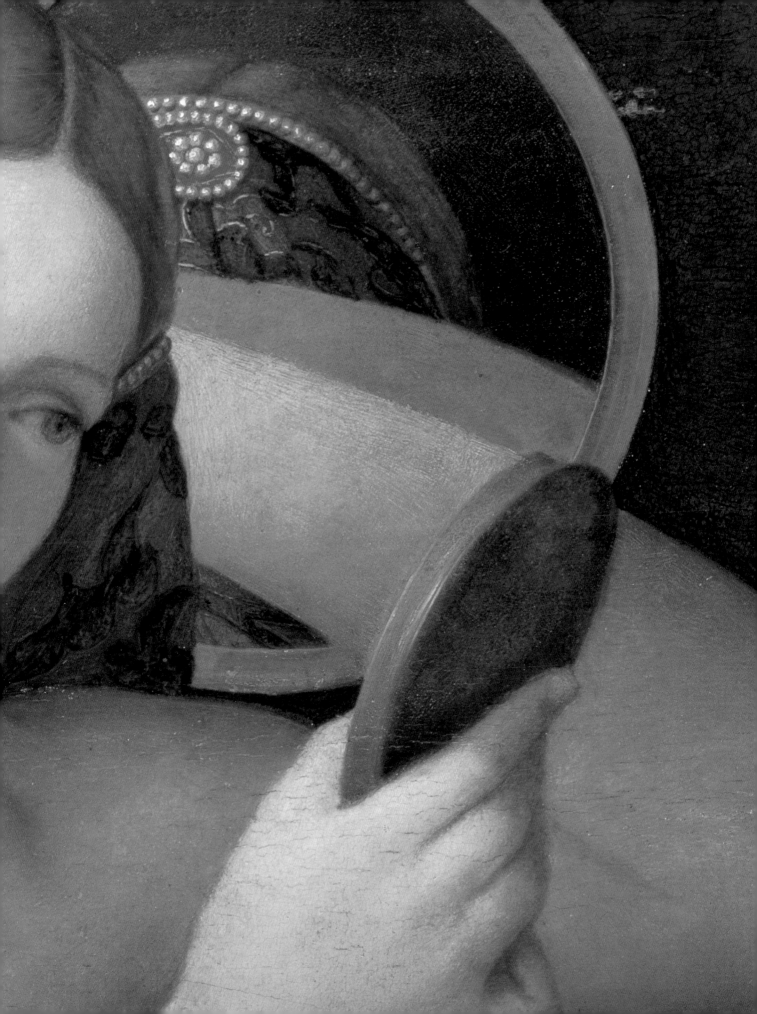

variation of the concept of placing the back hair in a bag – literally dressing it. Here, rather than employing the funnel or sausage seen in fig. 26, the hair is contained in a bag of lavish brocade material. At its mouth there is a band of pearls, secured, probably, by a drawstring at the nape of the neck. It is, presumably, U-shaped on the underside, to embrace the back of her head. In any event, the objective was surely to keep the hair hidden but flowing free within the bag, into which it is seen descending apparently effortlessly from the central parting above.

The result is extraordinarily sensual, with the girl apparently otherwise undressed, absorbed with her own image in a hand-held mirror. She is admiring the effect of the arrangement at the back of her head, reflected in a larger mirror to the rear. Frustratingly, her arm, holding the hair-bag in place, obscures most of its details. We can, however, see a large brooch in its centre just below the top, presumably hiding a pin passing through the hair itself. The fact that she is holding up the device with her hand suggests that the whole arrangement might all too easily slip to the floor, revealing her hair (and who would complain?) in all its glory. The sensuality of the picture comes to its climax when one reflects that here is a girl whose only visible item of clothing is covering the only part of her – her hair – which feels no cold, and which therefore surely needs no clothing other than to titillate the senses. It is the reverse, too, of the usual arrangement in which the top of the head is covered and the hair falls free beneath it. There is nothing to prevent cold wind or hot sunshine from reaching the girl's otherwise bare head. It is a splendid reversal of the usual, clearly as fascinating to

herself as it is to the painter and those of us who observe it all these centuries later. An advantage of such a bag (though surely not in this case) is that the wearer could convey to the observer the impression that she had voluminous hair hidden within it. In reality she might have no more than an appropriate amount of stuffing – an interesting alternative to hanging a hairpiece at the back of one's head.

During the late fifteenth century artist and hairdresser would seem to conspire to create increasingly fantastic hairstyles

In Spain in about 1500 the Duchess of Alba (fig. 30) wore her hair folded just below her ears and pulled back beneath a headdress, with a veil sweeping forwards across her breast. From the central parting, the front part of her hair is plaited to the left of her brow but appears to remain unplaited to the right. The hair behind the plait has been carefully waved. Here is a splendid balance between the natural and the contrived. Moving from Spain to Italy and from dark to blonde hair, at about the same time, the girl painted by Titian in fig. 31 likewise has her hair frizzed. It is loosely braided to the right of her forehead and tied back, like a curtain, around itself with gold braid. Titian clearly delighted in hair in the same way that Renoir was to do three centuries later. For Botticelli (fig. 32) that delight, though shared, would seem to be channelled into fascination with the complexities made possible by plaiting and interweaving. In fact, during the late fifteenth century artist and hairdresser would seem to conspire to create increasingly fantastic hairstyles, so that a girl's own mother could be excused for not knowing what was her daughter's own hair and what was not and, indeed,

PREVIOUS SPREAD:
FIG. 29. This girl wears her hair in a large brocade bag, contrasting with her own nakedness.
Giovanni Bellini, *Young Woman with a Mirror* (detail), 1515 (Kunsthistorisches Museum, Vienna)

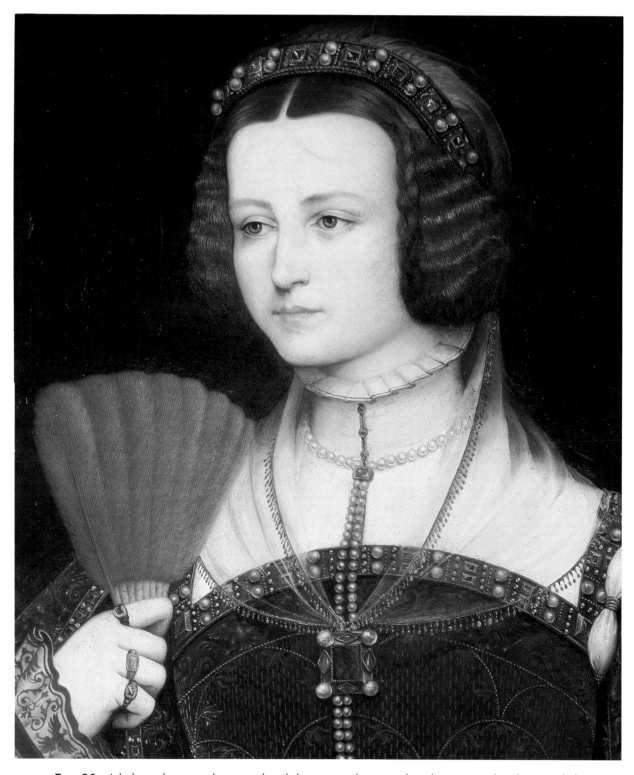

FIG. 30. A balance between the natural and the contrived — part plaited, part waved and part veiled.
Unknown artist, Isabel of Zuniga and Pimentel, daughter of the Duke of Arevalo, 2nd Duchess of Alba,
c.1500 (Collection of the Duke of Berwick and Alba, Madrid)

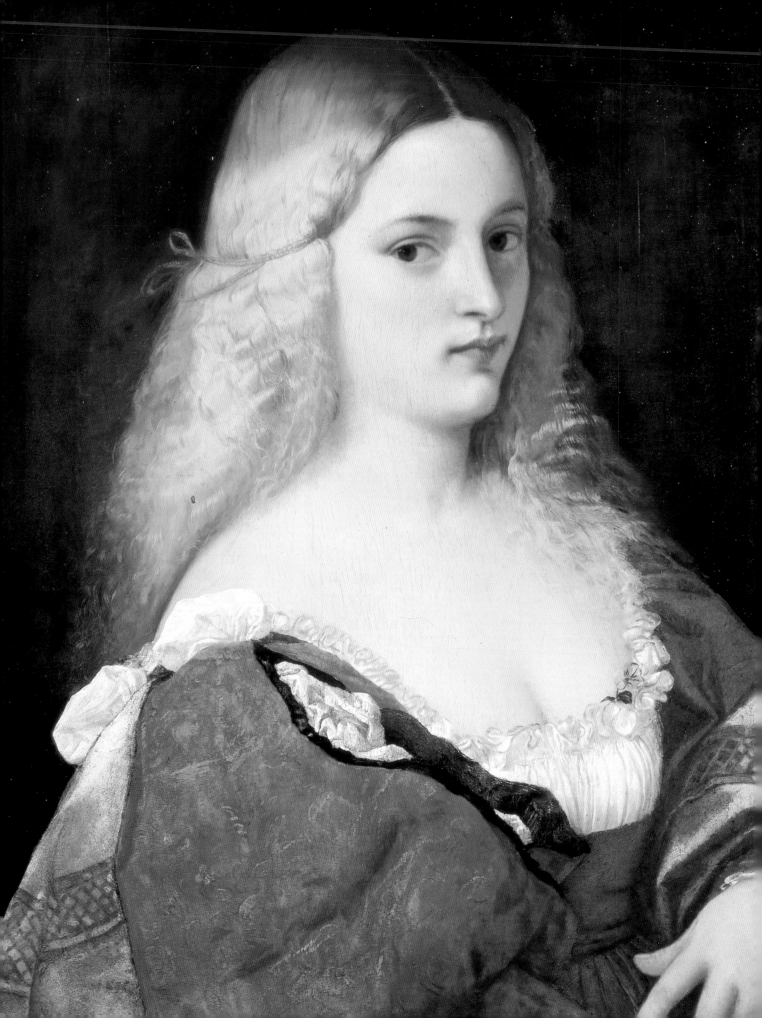

what was hair and what was material. The saving grace is that such styles were gorgeous rather than grotesque, the more usual outcome of a fashion taken to extreme.

Nonetheless, it is something of a relief to turn to the simplicity of the hairstyle of the 'Lady in Yellow' (fig. 33). However, on closer inspection this, too, proves somewhat complicated. She has a hairband looping her head from nape to brow as well as a brow band circling the top of her head. The hair is folded in tresses over both of these bands and the tresses themselves are interwoven. One tress is left to float down over the back of her neck and another to the side. Baldovinetti was no Raphael or Titian but, as a careful depicter of hairstyle, usefully presented in profile, he has done his job here both well and faithfully.

From the same period comes the timeless beauty of 'Flora' (fig. 34). With her hair centrally parted, carefully curled to either side of her head and gathered in a bun at the back, she could have come from Ancient Greece or Victorian England. She is testimony to the fact that, at any time, there is nothing to beat a beautiful woman with her hair simply dressed. But perhaps this is to read too much into matters concerning artistic influence and cross-border fashion, both in terms of space and time. There are only so many ways in which one can dress hair. The way in which it is dressed is probably more related to the time and the assistance available, and to the nature of the hair itself, than to the period.

Today we are concerned with a unified European monetary system; in Victorian times every royal house across Europe was related to Queen Victoria. But in the Renaissance period it was art that travelled quite as freely as commerce and blue blood. And, with art, travelled fashion. The point is that Europe, lacking today's speed of travel, nonetheless was an area through which fashion

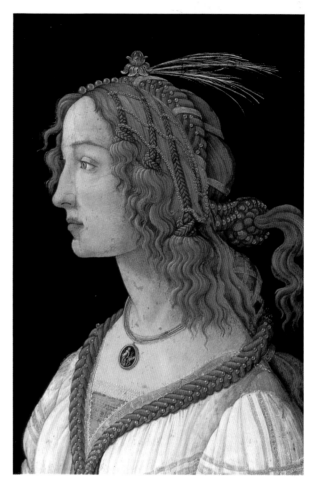

FIG. 32. The art of complexity – what is her own hair and what is not?
Sandro Botticelli, *Portrait of a Young Woman,* 1485 (Stadelsches Kunstinstitut, Frankfurt)

could filter assisted by art.

However, crossing the English Channel was another matter. It is a shock to realise that the young Elizabeth in fig. 35 is contemporary with the great Italian Renaissance seen at its height in figs 31 and 32. Perhaps we would think differently if she were painted by Titian or Botticelli rather than an unknown hand. As it is, she looks positively medieval. However, there has always been something retrospective about royalty. How else to emphasise continuity? If you are a queen, there is no need for an elaborate hairstyle – a crown is quite enough.

FIG. 31. A true Titian blonde with her hair frizzed and tied back like a curtain.
Tiziano Vecellio Titian, *Violante,* 1510–15 (Kunsthistorisches Museum, Vienna)

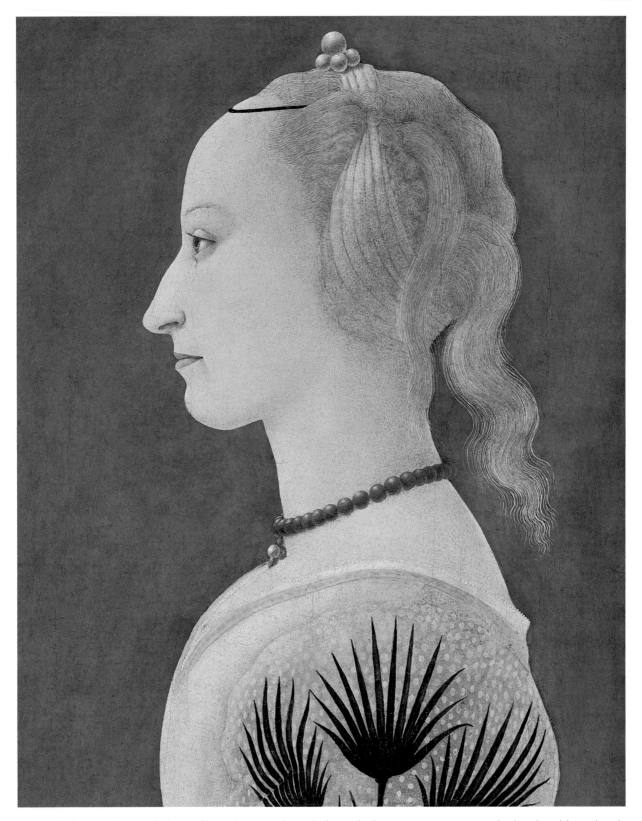

FIG. 33. Apparently simple but in fact rather complicated, this girl's hair is interwoven over the head and brow band. Alesso Baldovinetti, *Portrait of a Lady in Yellow*, probably 1465 (National Gallery, London)

Elizabeth wears her hair long and loose, its golden hue contrasting with the white of the ermine and merging with the gold of her cloak. She wears it so simply because this was the way in which a bride wore her hair at her marriage; likewise a queen at her coronation as she commits herself to her country. Elizabeth appears weighed down by the symbolism of monarchy in contrast to the simplicity of Princess Sybille of Cleves (fig. 19) with her equally natural hairstyle, as she approaches marriage, rather than monarchy, some fifty years before.

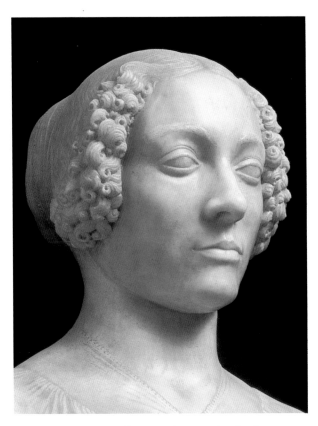

FIG. 34. Timeless simplicity – the flanking curls, central parting and bun could equally belong to Ancient Greece or Victorian England as to the Italian Renaissance.
Andrea del Verrocchio, *Young Woman with a Bunch of Flowers*, or *'Flora'*, marble bust, thought to be of Lucrezia Donati (detail), 1480s (Bargello, Florence)

The fact is that there are only so many ways in which one can dress hair. The way in which it is dressed is probably more related to the time and the assistance available, and to the nature of the hair itself, than to the period

It is a benefit of being neither rich nor famous that, if painted at all, you are generally only depicted when looking your most youthful and most beautiful. Not so with a great queen. We see Elizabeth again in fig. 36, in middle age, with her hair up and her forehead plucked. With jewels sewn into her hair, its complexity rivals that of her lace ruff. It is almost as if it is an article of clothing – in other words a wig – rather than her own hair. In all probability this is the case, because she did have a great number of wigs.

One young man of about the same time wore his own hair loose and long. This was Shakespeare's friend and patron, Henry Wriothesley, third Earl of Southampton. Elizabeth's father, Henry VIII, would not have approved. His male courtiers, like himself, were short-haired. However, this was a new age. The Renaissance had reached England, and new ages bring new hairstyles.

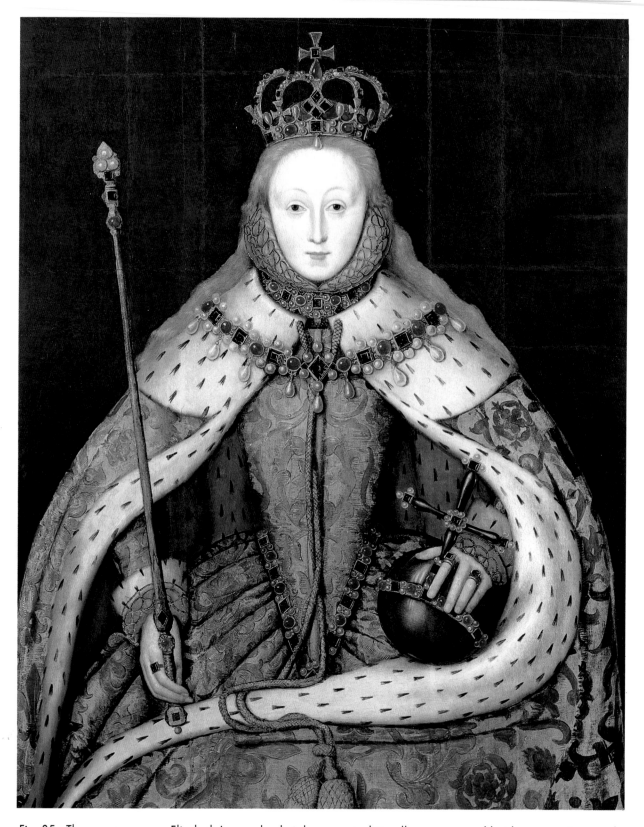

Fig. 35. The young queen — Elizabeth I wears her hair loose, as traditionally a queen would at her coronation, much like a bride at her marriage. Unknown artist, Elizabeth I (National Portrait Gallery, London)

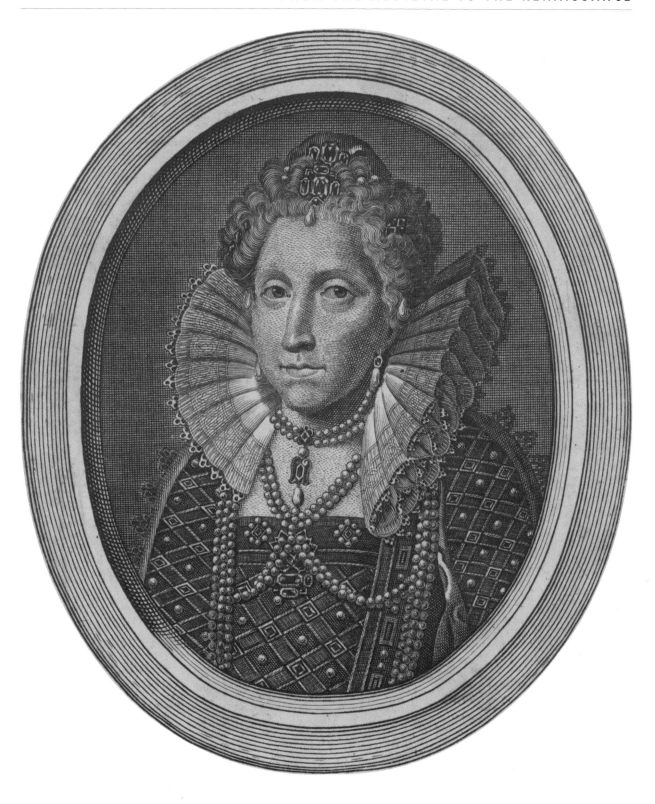

FIG. 36. The queen in middle age with her forehead plucked beneath what was probably a wig, used as a vehicle for impressive jewellery. Elizabeth I. Engraving by Antony Gucho after More (author's collection)

CAVALIERS, ROUNDHEADS AND PILGRIM FATHERS

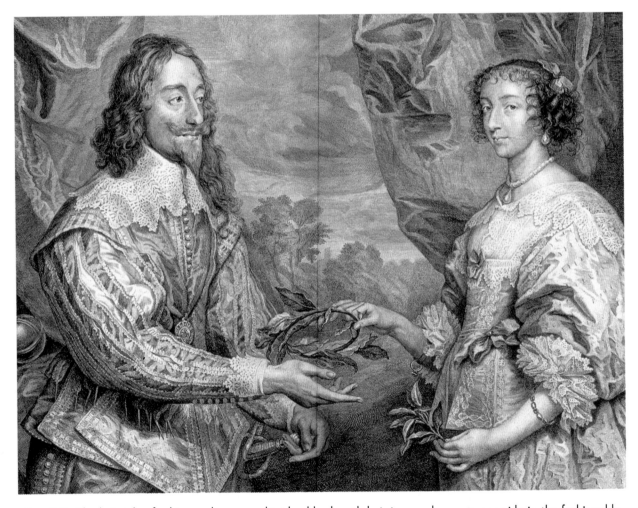

FIG. 37. The hairstyle of a king and queen — his shoulder-length hair is worn longer to one side in the fashionable 'lovelock', while she has a fringe and 'confidants' hanging over her ears, making her look rather like a spaniel, a breed forever associated with the Stuarts.
Charles I (1600—49) and Henrietta Maria (1609—69), 1742 engraving by George Vertue from a 1634 painting after Van Dyck (private collection)

It is extraordinary that something as superficial as hair should so decisively define groups of people, right to the core of their faith and their politics. However, this is the case. As good an example as any is that of the Cavaliers and Roundheads. Less typically, with them it is the male hairstyle, rather than the female, which is the focus of attention. The Cavalier one envisages as mounted on his horse with hair flowing to beneath the shoulder; the Roundhead one perceives as an infantryman, with the shorter haircut that earned him the name Roundhead.

At the forefront of the Cavaliers comes Charles I, Scottish, with papal leanings, and with a French wife, Henrietta Maria. Together they brought high fashion to the English court. In their double portrait (fig. 37) it is for once the husband at whom one looks first. It is Charles's own hair that falls to his right shoulder and is seen, to the fore, well below the shoulder on his left side. This longer piece of hair is his highly fashionable 'lovelock', or 'cadenette', a splendid affectation that originated in France. It was first adopted by Honoré d'Albert, Maréchal de France, who was also Señor de Cadenet (hence 'cadenette'). Unlike Charles I, he had not just one but two cadenettes, falling forward over both shoulders. These can be seen to this day (but not much longer if the lawyers have their way) in the full-bottomed wig of a judge, longer at the front than it is at the back. However, the asymmetry of Charles's single lovelock is surely more stylish. The ladies certainly thought so, since they widely copied it.

There is something charming about the lovelock's appearance in this double portrait. This is because a lovelock was rather like the 'favour' that a knight would wear in honour of the object of his love. However, rather than wearing her glove or some such token in his helmet, instead the man demonstrates his affection by leaving a part of his hair to grow longer than the rest. It is as if he is so engrossed in his regard for his lady that he has absentmindedly forgotten to have his hair cut evenly, leaving the chair before the barber has completed his ministrations, so impatient is he to be with her.

Charles' hair is seen to even better effect in the famous Van Dyck triple portrait (fig. 38) painted for

The ringlets, cruches and confidants all required careful attention, usefully from the maid but sometimes from the lady herself

Bernini. The love lock is still more clearly seen, but without the bow on that sported by Edward Sackville some years before (fig. 39).

And the object of Charles's affections? There she is on the other side of the picture. His hair is down and flowing free, whereas hers is demurely bunched above the nape of her neck. Unlike him, she has a fringe above her forehead, carefully set in individual curls or 'cruches'. Over her ears hang longer curls or 'confidants'. Not only does she bring to London the hairstyle of the French court but she also brings the vocabulary to go with it.

These confidants give Henrietta Maria something of the appearance of a spaniel with its curly-coated ears. In fact, one breed of that very dog was to be so favoured by her elder son (also Charles) that it came to be known in time as the King Charles Spaniel. It is interesting to speculate whether the Stuarts favoured the spaniel because it reminded them of their womenfolk. Alternatively, did their wives dress their hair to echo the appearance of this favourite breed of dog?

OVERLEAF:

FIG. 38. This sculptor's guide could equally assist the hairdresser. Charles I, W. Sharp after Van Dyck (author's collection)

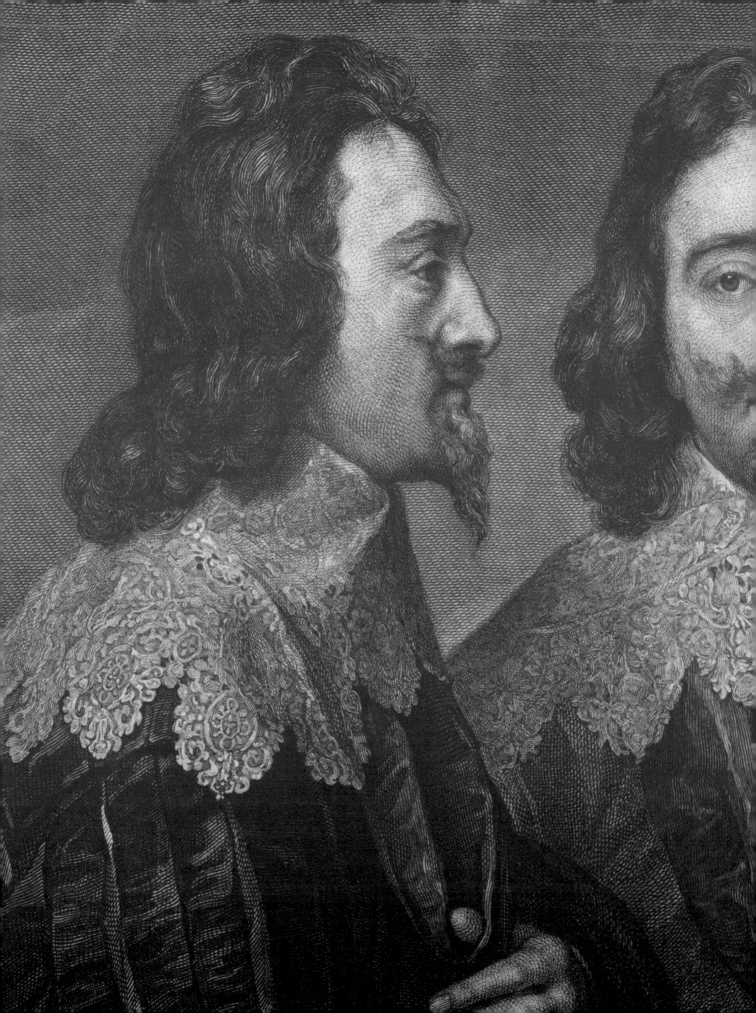

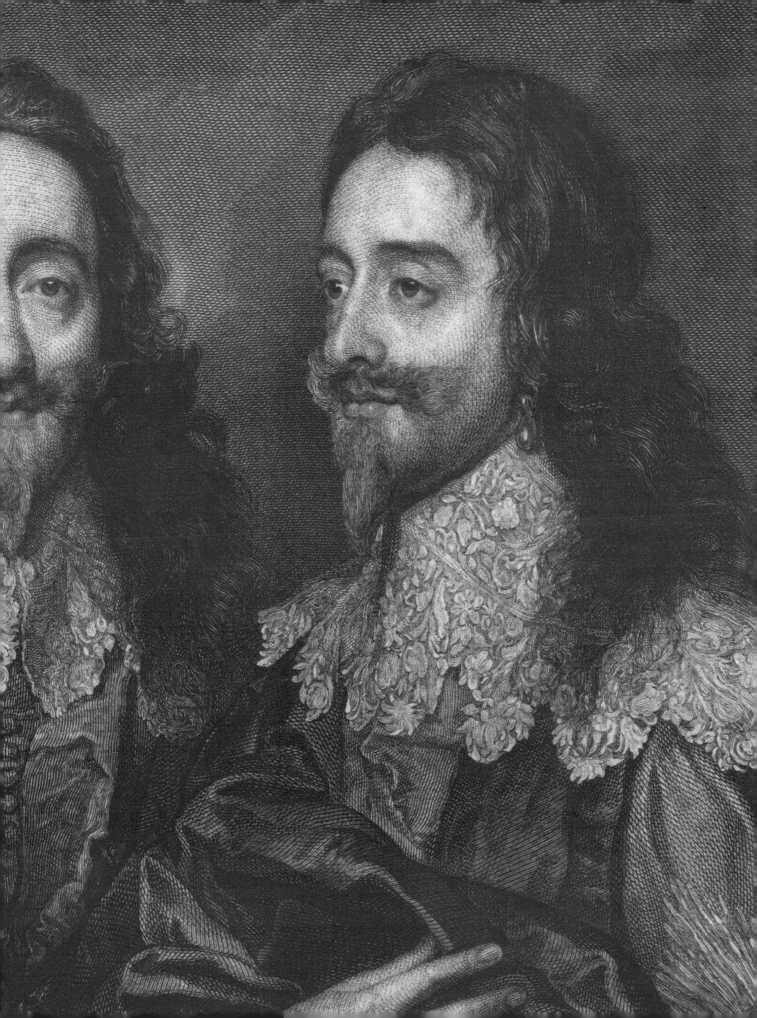

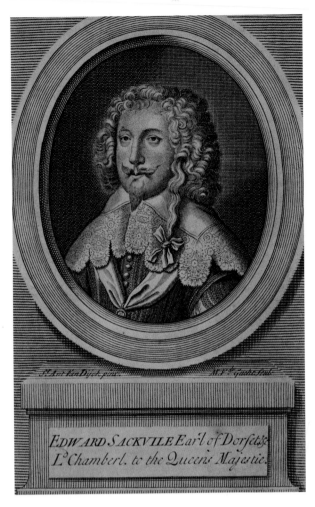

J. Ant. van Dyck, pinx.   *M. V. Guche, Sculp.*

EDWARD SACKVILE Earl of Dorset &c. Ld Chamberl. to the Queen's Majestie.

FIG. 39. Lovelock complete with bow. *Edward Sackville*, Guche after Van Dyck (author's collection)

The children of this particular happy marriage are shown in fig. 40. On the left is Mary, here aged six, whose hairstyle and dress echo those of her mother. Next to her is her brother, four-year-old James, still in petticoats, a reminder that long hair and petticoats on a young boy was the traditional way of disguising the male child, lest he be carried off by the devil. Proudly in the centre stands the seven-year-old Charles, who was to have a breed of a spaniel named after him. Just as his eldest sister's hair and dress echo those of her mother, so do those of his father, with his spreading lace collar setting off his dark tresses. There is even the hint of a lovelock in the way that it lies forward upon his left shoulder but not upon his right, though one suspects that this was no more than a suggestion. The hair is perhaps simply the same length all round, with that to the right of him being tossed back, and that to the left just happening to fall forward. A lovelock would surely be rather too sophisticated to be adopted by a young boy. Charles's splendid dog (not in this case a spaniel) takes up much of the remainder of the picture, but there is still room for two-year-old Elizabeth, being terribly grown-up with one-year-old Anne. So far as we can see, Anne has little or no hair to speak of, but Elizabeth has hers protruding in a fringe beneath her cap. In this respect alone all the older children reflect the hairstyle of their mother, rather than their father. The fringe, though perhaps rather effeminate, was presumably deemed more practical for a child who might not be trusted to keep hair out of eyes and mouth.

Effeminate or not, the fringe was favoured by that greatest of all the Roundheads, Oliver Cromwell (fig. 41). Like master, like servant – we see that the boy who is attending to the sash around his waist likewise has a fringe. What is intriguing is that the remainder of their hair is not significantly shorter than that of King Charles, executed at the beginning of that year. It is perhaps a myth that the English Civil War was a battle between the long- and the short-haired. The Roundheads could perhaps more appropriately have been called the 'Fringeheads'. However, style is as much related to authority as it is to taste. Here is Cromwell, no longer the revolutionary leader but the Lord Protector, having his official portrait painted, not on this occasion 'warts and all', but in a manner supposed to be reassuringly regal to those royalists now forced to recognise his rule. If they could see him as a civilised gentleman rather than a rabble-rouser, so much the better, and a civilised hairstyle, as any public relations man will tell you, is an essential element in the politician's armoury. The same criterion applies to Cromwell's daughter, Elizabeth Claypole (fig. 42). She has neither the 'cruches', curls on the forehead, nor the 'confidants', clusters of curls over the ears, favoured by Henrietta Maria, but she does have ringlets, which frame her neck and shoulders becomingly. She must have appeared reassuringly civilised to a royalist coming to terms with living under the new regime.

Queen or commoner, however, a civilised, sophisticated appearance comes at a price. The ringlets, cruches and confidants all required careful attention, usually from the maid but sometimes from the lady herself. Be it France, England or Holland, a lady's care and concern for her hair and the way in which she dressed were much the same, certainly at this time of civil war and traffic to and fro across the Channel and the North Sea. Style was much less important for those who journeyed further across the Atlantic. The Pilgrim Fathers had landed in America twenty-nine years before the Nonconformist Cromwell would have made their life in England more attractive. The austerity in terms of fashion and their dislike of decoration means that – as in biblical times with the commandment against making graven images – they left little record behind them. Accordingly we have to rely on later reconstructions, such as those which show Anne Hutchinson preaching in her house in Boston in 1637. Her head is invariably shown as covered so that her hair is only visible at the brow band. The heads of all her female listeners are likewise shown as covered. The men who listen to her would have been scandalised were it

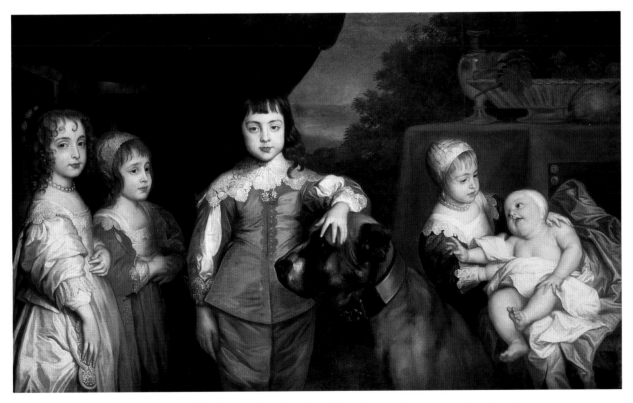

FIG. 40. Royal children – shoulder-length hair for the boys and ringlets for the girls; fringes for all except the baby. Unknown artist, after Van Dyck, *Five Children of Charles I*, 1637

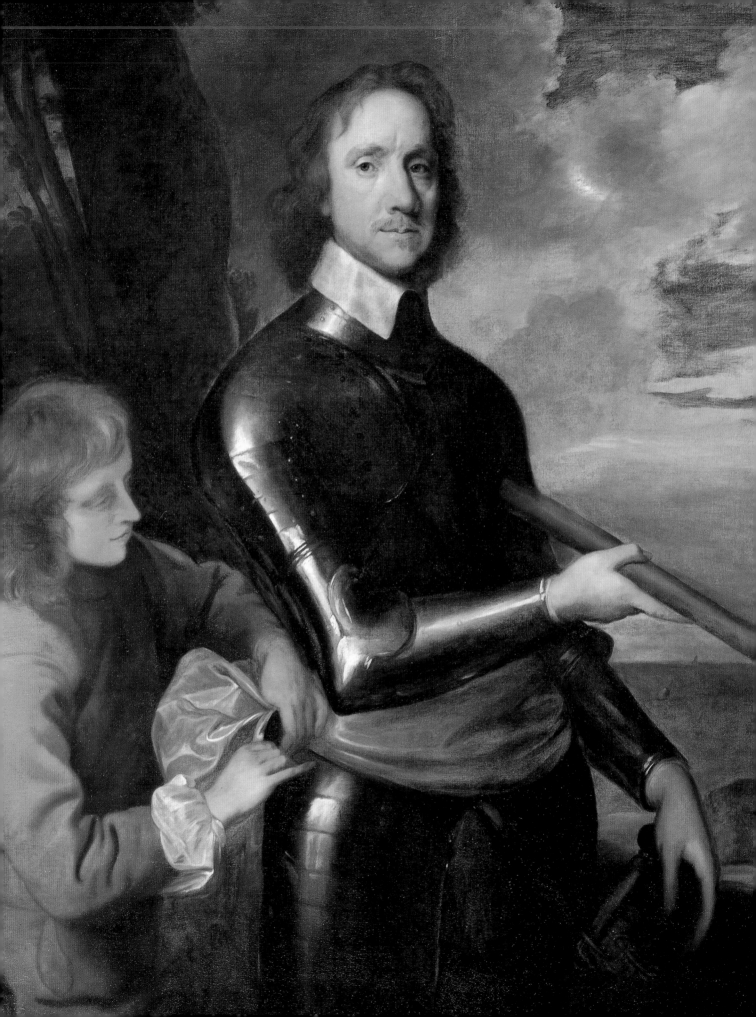

Be it France, England or Holland, a lady's care and concern for her hair and the way in which she dressed were much the same

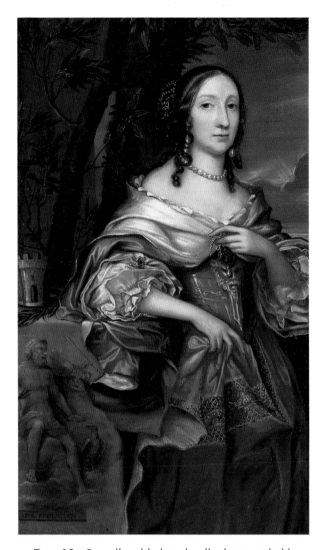

otherwise. One wonders if the male desire to keep the female head so fully covered was entirely motivated by the concept that the bible requires women to be modest. There must surely have also been something of the husband's wish to ensure that only he could see his wife's 'crowning glory', and that in the privacy of the bedchamber.

Men were, however, not so strict about their own appearance, with flowing locks often evident beneath their large hats, as we see in imaginary images depicting the signing of the treaty with the Indians or the Pilgrim Fathers' first landing. Such pictures, incidentally, also often feature native Americans in the background, some sporting a hairstyle which, much later, would travel the other way across the Atlantic – the Mohican.

The emphasis on outward appearance and show from which the Pilgrim Fathers had fled was to be banished from their native England for the eleven years of the Commonwealth. However, extravagant fashion was shortly to be restored to popularity, returning across the North Sea and English Channel, richer and more varied than ever before.

FIG. 42. Roundhead lady – hardly distinguishable from her Cavalier counterpart, Oliver Cromwell's daughter has her face framed becomingly with ringlets, though most Roundhead ladies would have had their heads covered.
John Michael Wright, *Elizabeth Claypole*, 1658 (National Portrait Gallery, London)

FIG. 41. Roundhead gentleman – contrary to popular belief, Roundhead men wore their hair hardly shorter than did the Cavaliers, but here Cromwell, unlike the usurped king, has a fringe, as does his page.
Robert Walker, *Oliver Cromwell*, c.1649 (National Portrait Gallery, London)

RESTORATION TO REVOLUTION:

EXTREMES OF FASHION IN THE SEVENTEENTH AND EIGHTEENTH CENTURIES

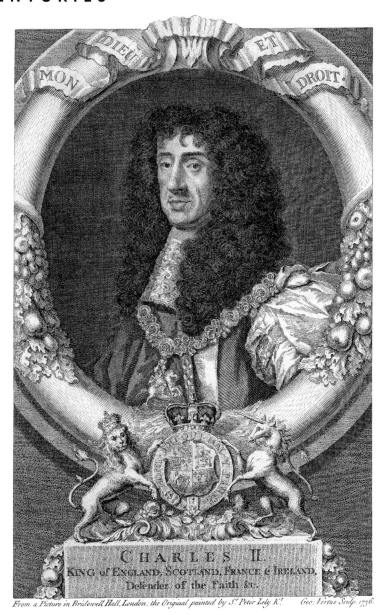

FIG. 43. Long but false – following the newly established French fashion, Charles II wore a wig, longer than his own hair when he was a boy.
Engraving by George Vertue (?)
(author's collection)

The Stuarts from England sought refuge at the French court. At its centre was Louis XIV, who boasted an abundance of his own splendid hair. However, he found himself increasingly outshone by his courtiers, who wore ever more sumptuous wigs over their shaven heads. Finally, in 1662, he too consented to having his head shaved. Charles II, the King in Exile (last seen as a small boy with his hand on his dog in fig. 41), kept his own naturally black hair until it began to turn grey. It was then that he too succumbed to the wearing of a wig. Accordingly, he appears in fig. 43, having been restored to his throne in 1660, sporting dark hair, but not his own. Indeed, it is far more sumptuous than ever were his father's own natural locks. From the court of Versailles, English ladies in exile were also to catch a glimpse of the beginnings of more extravagant coiffure. Spanish ladies were likewise to be influenced by these new fashions when Maria Theresa, daughter of Philip IV of Spain, became queen to Louis XIV.

One of the more dramatic of these new styles was the 'hurluberlu', which first appeared in 1671. It involved a riot of curls over the head but with locks of straight hair, twisted at the tips, flowing down from below the curls to cover the shoulders. Another elaborate style was the 'fontange', said to have originated from an incident out hunting, when the Duchesse de Fontange's hair came down. With great presence of mind, she bound it up with a garter. The king was enchanted. The tale is the more poignant because the duchess died shortly after at the age of twenty, but the style that she had created went from strength to strength, becoming more and more elaborate and ridiculous. The king grew heartily to dislike the style, which held sway until Lady Sandwich (fig. 44) came to the court from England. When the king openly admired her much simpler hair arrangement, the ladies at court quickly took note – a rare example of fashion moving from England to France, rather than vice versa.

Back in England, Charles II was enchanted by Nell Gwyn. Early portraits show her as having a happily abandoned mixture of hair partly up and partly down. She was, however, to replace such simplicity with ringlets

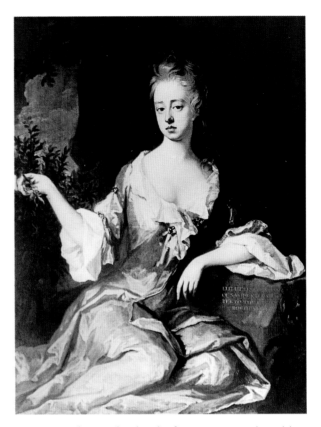

FIG. 44. The Sandwich? The fontange was eclipsed by the much simpler style of Lady Sandwich when she visited the court of Versailles from England.
Michael Dahl, *Elizabeth, 3rd Countess of Sandwich* (Birmingham Museums & Art Gallery) with thanks to the Earl of Sandwich for locating it

after 1669. Whereas men found the truly female enchanting, women derived a certain frisson from adopting male styles. If men could shave their heads and wear elaborate wigs, then women would do likewise, openly rather than furtively. It was just one step further actually to adopt an enigmatically masculine appearance. Henrietta Cavendish (fig. 45) is just such a tease, seen here in her tricorn hat and neck cloth or stock. Only the skirt beneath her riding coat gives the game away. And if one is having one's hair cut or shaved to be hidden

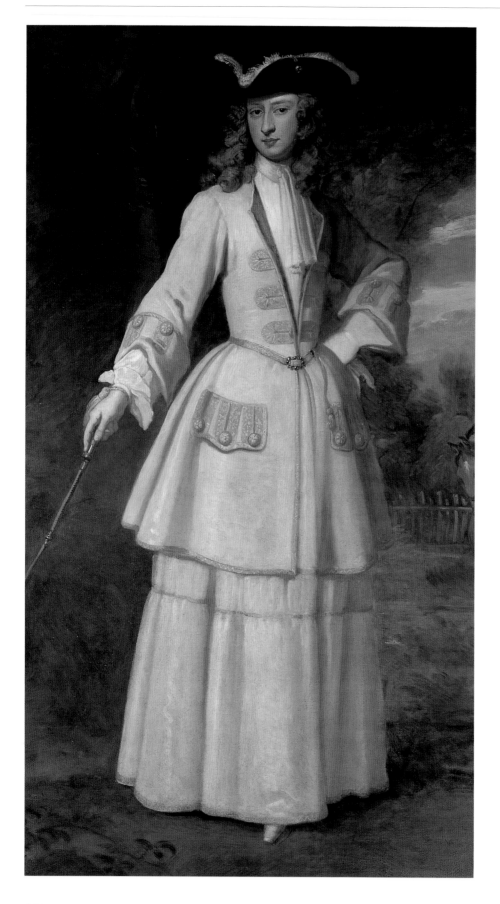

FIG. 45. Wearing male plumage – a man's wig can look equally stylish on a woman. Sir Godfrey Kneller, *Henrietta Cavendish, Lady Huntingdon,* seventeenth century (Ham House, Surrey)

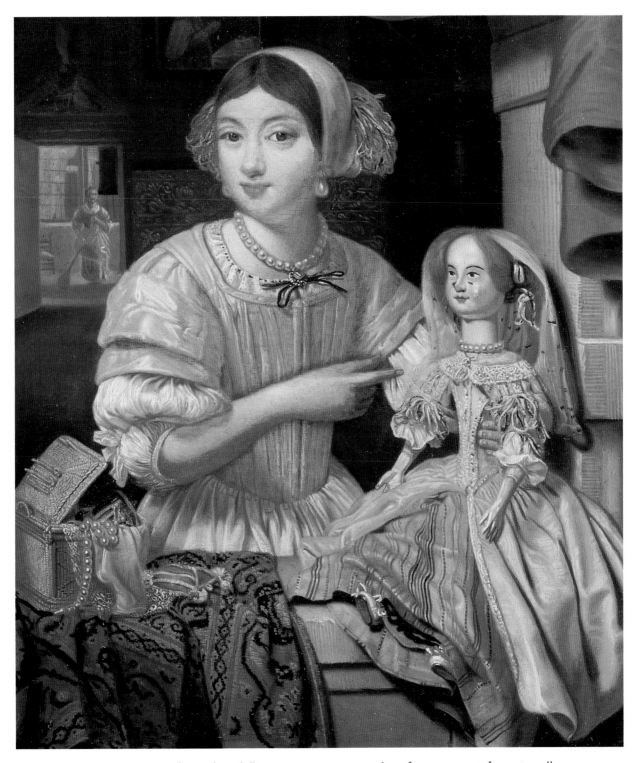

FIG. 46. Not just to play with – dolls were an important medium for conveying information all over Europe concerning the latest hair and dress styles.
Edwaert Colyer or Collier, *Young Woman Holding a Doll in an Interior with a Maid Sweeping Behind*
(Johnny van Haeften Gallery, London)

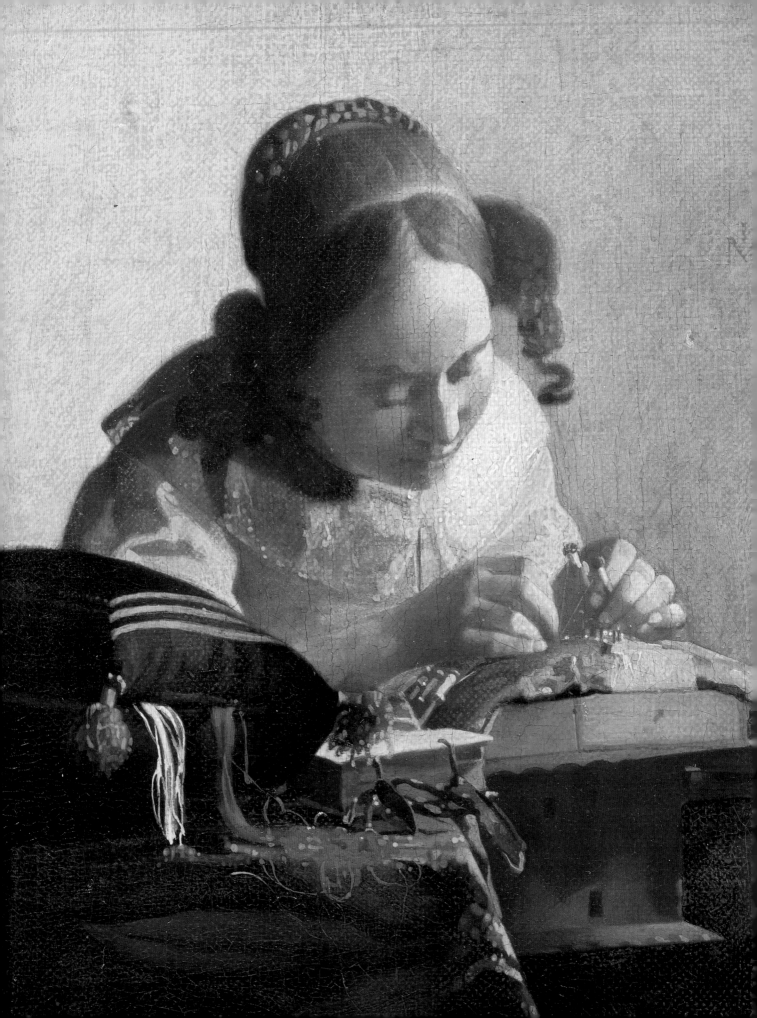

beneath a wig, why not wear one's own hair naturally, cut relatively short like a boy's? You could always cover it up again with a wig. Artifice is everything.

Through paintings and via travel between courts, fashion would spread from country to country. There was also another important medium – the doll. The girl in fig. 46 is not so much playing with her doll as using it to demonstrate different hairstyles and clothing. Dolls were sent all over Europe for this very purpose. For instance, Madame de Sévigné sent one to her daughter with the hair made up in the new 'hurluberlu' style. Today's Barbie doll with her changes of clothing, hairstyles and now even tattoos, has a long and cosmopolitan ancestry.

Many a peasant, all over Europe, would simply be growing her hair in a long plait, ready for it to be harvested for the wig market. However, it was not just the gentry and aristocracy who were permitted a certain pride in their hairstyle, as can be seen in the view of the little lacemaker captured at her work by Jan Vermeer (fig. 47). This master of the Dutch interior depicts the lacemaker's hairstyle with equal faithfulness. The girl's inclined head gives us the opportunity to see better than she ever could every detail of her coiffure. There is the central parting at the front, with the front hair worn in ringlets to either side, and pulled back to the ear. Then there is the parting of the back hair, from ear to ear across the head. Finally, it is wound together at the back within an encircling plait. Equally enchanting was a simpler contemporary arrangement of hair pulled back evenly from the forehead, again to an encircling plait.

Simpler still was the style where the hair was pulled back in what would now be called a ponytail. Then it would have been called a 'queue' and is more likely to have been seen on a man than a woman. Such a man

Fig. 47. T-junction – the way in which her hair is parted is clearly seen in the inclined head of this girl at work. Jan Vermeer, *The Lacemaker*, 1669–70 (Louvre Museum, Paris)

was Charles Edward Stuart, alias Bonnie Prince Charlie (fig. 48), here drawn ten years or so before his ill-fated return from the French court to Scotland. He took flight 'over the sea to Skye' with the redoubtable Flora Macdonald (fig. 49), whose relatively shorter hair, carefully curled for the artist, shows the practical girl that she was. Was she perhaps just a little amused to have Charles disguised as her French lady's maid? The disguise must surely have been relatively easy with his hair, if anything, longer than hers.

Through paintings and via travel between courts, fashion would spread from country to country. There was also another important medium – the doll

Lest it be thought that American life was all Puritan gloom, fig. 50 proves otherwise. Mrs John Vinal poses in 1748 as sumptuously clad as Flora Macdonald, her contemporary, and has a similarly simple and becoming hairstyle. Clearly, if one were sufficiently far away from London or Paris, elegance and good sense could prevail. These qualities are hardly evident, however, in the lady of 1755 seen in fig. 51. She is typical of the many women of the time, both in London and Paris, who indulged in such extravagant hair constructions. They would either wear wigs or tease their own hair around pads and wired structures, topping the lot, as here, with some extraordinary hat. The whole concoction would have to stay in place for weeks on end, so there would be ample opportunity for vermin to find comfortable accommodation within the structure. It would also be liberally sprayed with powder to make it appear to be white. Whereas Charles II had favoured black hair, now, in the middle of the eighteenth century, white hair was all the rage for both young and old – gratifyingly so for

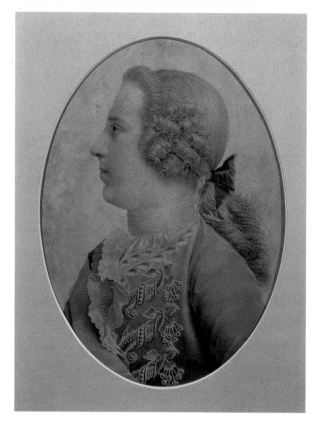

FIG. 48. The pretender to the Scottish throne, sporting his 'queue'.
Giles Hussey, *Portrait of Charles Edward Stuart*, alias 'Bonnie Prince Charlie', c.1735
(Philip Mould, Historical Portraits Ltd, London)

The eighteenth and nineteenth centuries saw thousands of jobs spring up in hairdressing and wig-making that had never existed before

scene, but the lady is having to sit in her peignoir to protect her clothes from powder from her coiffure. Her hairdresser is working painstakingly at her back and the proceedings are obviously taking a very long time, hence the book on her knee. This picture conveys another aspect of that extraordinary stuff called hair, in that lucrative trades can be built around its care and maintenance. The eighteenth and nineteenth centuries saw thousands of jobs spring up in hairdressing and wig-making that had never existed before.

As the century wore on, the powdered hair remained but the absurd styles subsided. Gainsborough and Reynolds had always refused to paint them, preferring to portray their sitters in a simpler, more timeless, classical style rather than some up-to-the-minute aberration of fashion. They argued that both they and their subjects would thus be better served by posterity – and how right they were. Thus it was that Reynolds portrayed the Hornecks sisters with very simple hairstyles (fig. 54), the one in profile and the other nearly full

the latter. Did Charles later come to regret shaving his head, one wonders, just because it had begun to go grey? Perhaps he should have waited.

Be that as it may, all this extremism in hair fashion provided a good subject for caricature. However, in truth one cannot be sure to what extent, because the styles and the methods of achieving them were so extreme as almost to defy exaggeration. Fig. 52 shows a man in his powder closet having powder wafted across his head by his valet. He holds a mask in front of his nose that looks, for all the world, like the 'drop snout' at the front end of Concorde. Fig. 53 shows a slightly less turbulent

FIG. 49. Relatively short and carefully curled – a no-nonsense saviour of a prince.
Allan Ramsay, *Portrait of Flora Macdonald*
(Ashmolean Museum, Oxford)

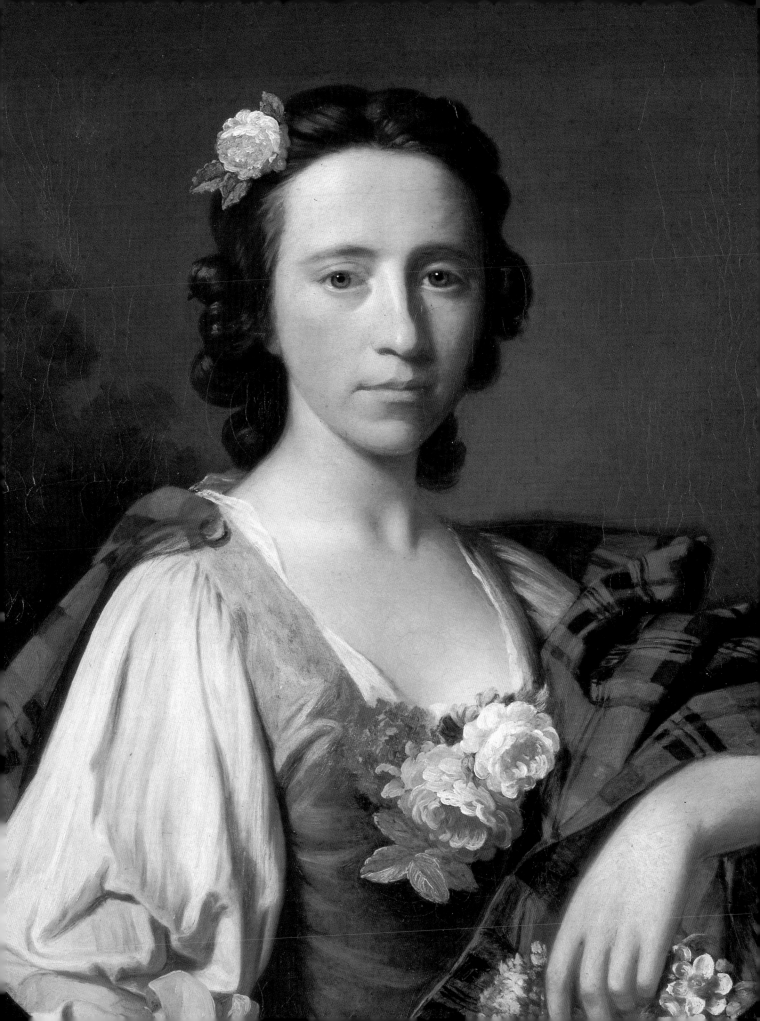

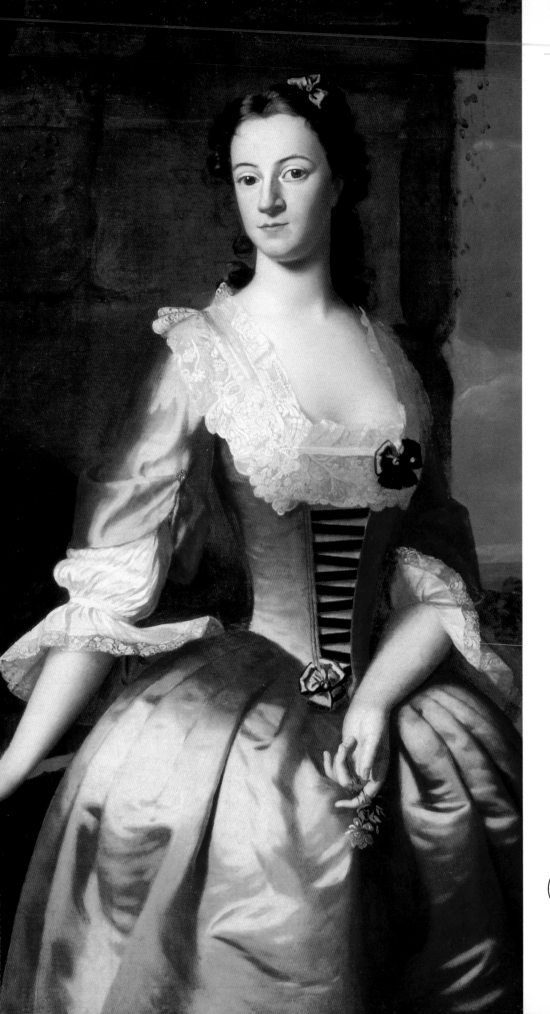

FIG. 50. American colonial elegance. Robert Feke, *Portrait of Mrs John Vinal*, 1748 (Brooklyn Museum of Art, New York)

Whereas Charles II had favoured black hair, now, in the middle of the eighteenth century, white hair was all the rage for both young and old

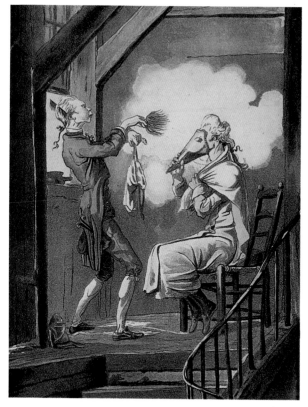

FIG. 52. Powder came with the craze for white hair and would be applied in a choking cloud in ones powder closet. *The toilet of an Attorney's Clerk*, eighteenth-century engraving by P. L. Debucourt after Antoine Charles Vernet (private collection)

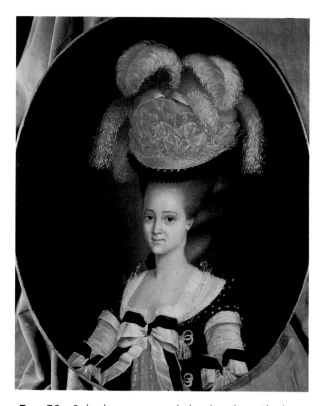

FIG. 51. Ridiculous extremes led to hair being built up over pads (often harbouring vermin) and topped with an amazing bonnet, fashionable in England and France. J. Mulnier, *Portrait of a Lady in a Hat*, c.1755 (Rafael Valls Gallery, London)

face. They could almost be one and the same person, but that one has her pearls round her neck and the other binding her hair.

However, (perhaps if the sitter was grand enough) Reynolds could be prevailed upon to paint a newly fashionable style. In fig. 55 we see the Duchess of Devonshire sporting the 'hedhehog' style, bouffant on top with trailing locks behind.

To balance the sexes, fig. 56 shows small boys of the period. The happy trio are Lord Melbourne's sons. The baby is in petticoats and (it would seem) his mother's hat. His elder brothers are in breeches and all three have

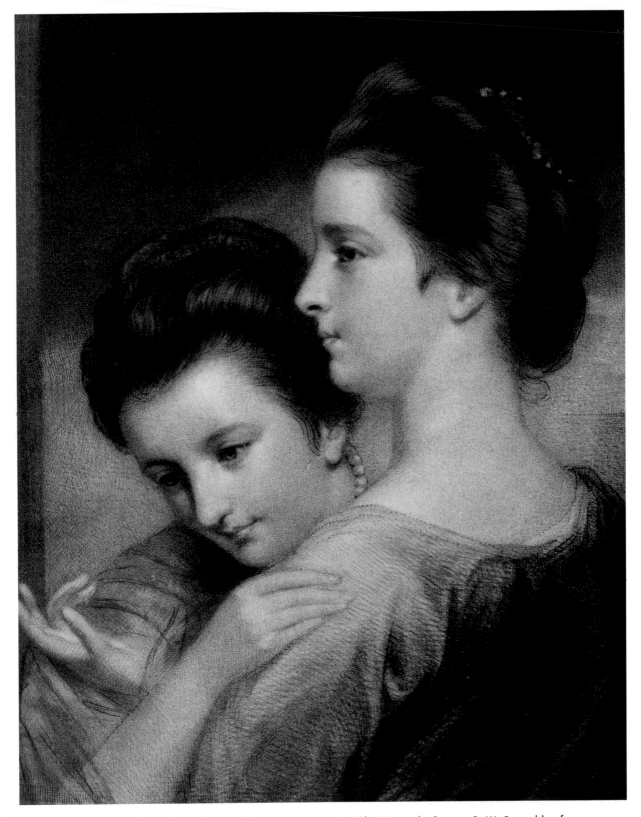

FIG. 54. A classical simplicity with an eye to posterity. *The Hornecks Sisters,* S .W. Reynolds after Sir Joshua Reynolds (author's collection)

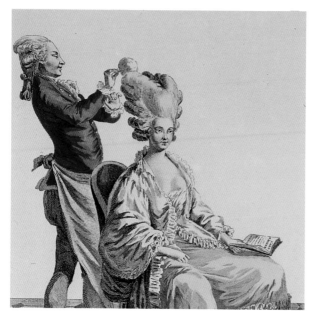

very practical fringes and shoulder length hair.

Fig. 57 shows a fine American lady wearing an elaborate powdered wig. However, it is in the style of none other than the 'hurluberlu' that hit Paris just under a century before. Is she behind the times in this respect, or is she confusing us by deliberately dressing out of period?

Boucher's wonderful study of the back of a girl's head from the eighteenth century (fig. 58) is elegantly timeless. Marie Antoinette was synonymous with the impending revolution that was to bring all this style and glamour to a halt. She played her own part in this trend towards simplicity, however. Her own hair, as a result of childbirth, became much thinner. Accordingly she adopted simpler styles and her courtiers did likewise.

FIG. 53 A lady's shoulders had to be protected from the powder by a 'peignoir' while her hairdresser made the finishing touches.
A Young Woman in a Peignoir with her Hairdresser, 1778 engraving by Dupin after Pierre Thomas Le Clerc (private collection)

FIG. 55. Fashion for the moment – hedgehog by name and hedgehog by nature. *The Duchess of Devonshire and Lady G. Cavendish,* S.W. Reynolds after Sir Joshua Reynolds (author's collection)

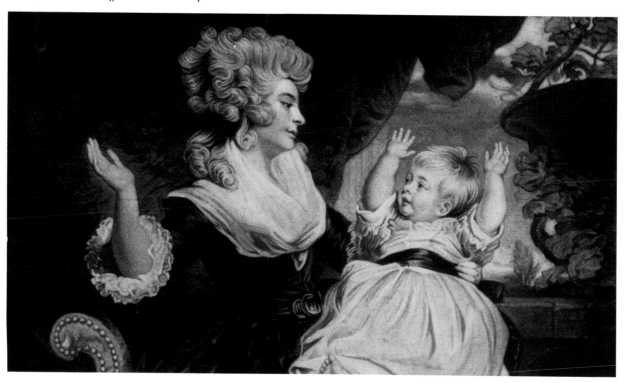

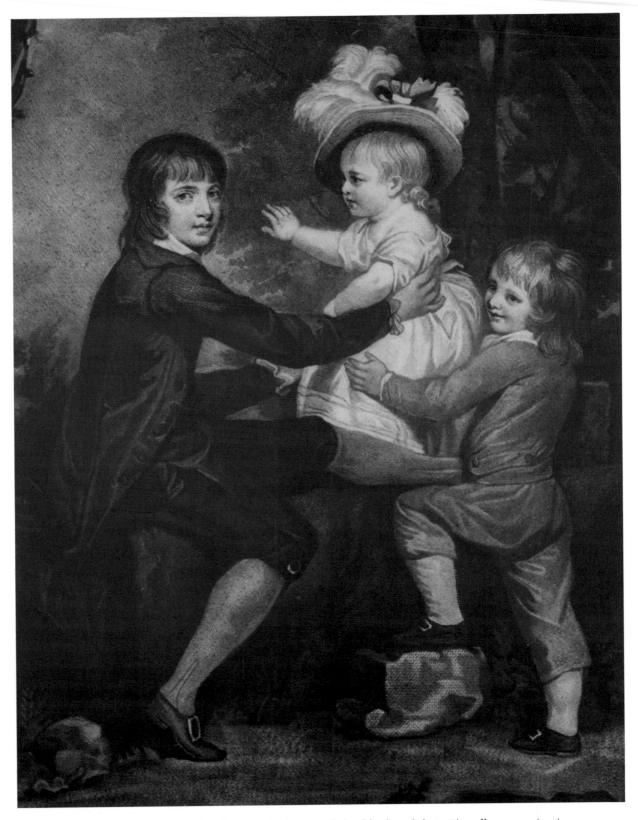

FIG. 56. Boys of the period with practical fringes and shoulder length hair. *The affectionate brothers,*
S.W. Reynolds after Sir Joshua Reynolds (author's collection).

This reduced show was, of course, hardly likely to halt the tumbrels and the guillotine – not that it was ever intended to do so. However, it did perhaps mark the century's final swing, in terms of hair style, between excess and elegance.

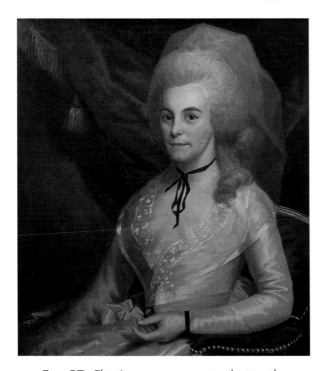

FIG. 57. This American women is adopting the 'hurluberlu' of the previous century.
Ralph Earl or Earle, *Portrait of Elizabeth Schuyler Hamilton, Wife of Alexander Hamilton*, late eighteenth century (Museum of the City of New York)

FIG. 58. Simpler elegance – this study shows how Marie Antoinette's hair might have been dressed when it became less abundant after childbirth.
François Boucher, *Head of a Girl from Behind*, eighteenth century (Christie's Images, London)

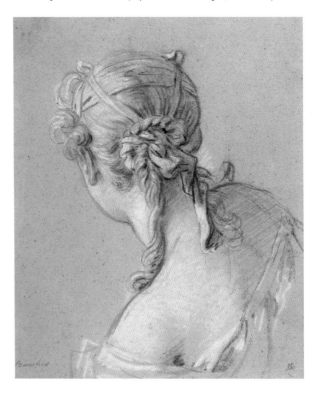

REVOLUTIONARY HAIRSTYLES:

THE AMERICAN WAR OF INDEPENDENCE, THE FRENCH REVOLUTION AND THE NAPOLEONIC WARS

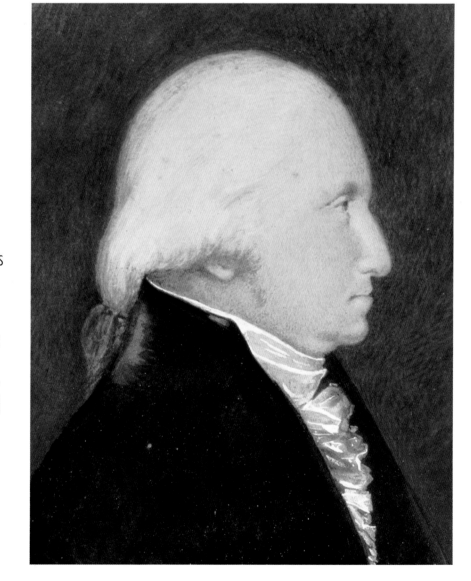

FIG. 59 The first president with powdered hair as long as a king's.
George Washington (1732–99), First President of the United States (1789–97), painted by a niece of General Lee after James Sharples (Chateau de Versailles, France/Roger-Viollet, Parsi)

As with the civil war in England, so with revolution and war in France and America, one turns first to look at male rather than female hair.

George Washington (fig. 59) has his hair tied in a queue, and adorned with quite as much powder as might be found upon the wig of his adversary, George III. Before the revolution he wore it equally long, but unpowdered. In 1780 he required that all soldiers should have their hair combed and powdered on parade and observed that 'to wear the hair cut or tied in the same manner throughout a whole corps would … be a very considerable ornament'. So it is today, although armies now aspire to achieve a uniform shortness, rather than a uniform length.

America's third president, Thomas Jefferson (fig. 60), wore his own hair throughout his life parted simply and falling to just below the shoulder. The style was much like that of the great royalist, Charles I, and the great republican, Oliver Cromwell. This is indicative that it is often character, rather than fashion or political leaning, that is the true determinant of an individual's hairstyle. Jefferson was nothing if not an individual.

These two American presidents, co-founders of a new nation, consciously cultivated a sense of continuity and respectability, in the same way as that other revolutionary, Oliver Cromwell, had been anxious to appear reassuringly civilised.

Napoleon was another matter. The French Revolution called not for continuity in style, but for change. Nowhere was that change more evident than in the evolution of Napoleon's own hairstyle. As a cadet at his

military academy he wore his hair in a queue and his position could be identified by the colour of the bow with which it was tied. By the time he was a young commander, he was wearing his hair loose to just below

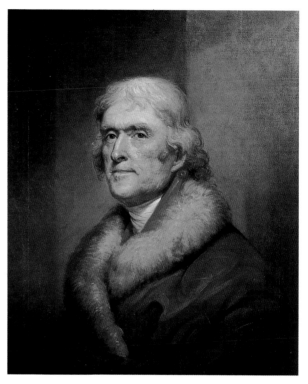

FIG. 60. Hair loose to the shoulders and no nonsense with powder.
Rembrandt Peale, *Thomas Jefferson (1743–1826), Third President of the United States, 1805*
(New York Historical Society)

> **America's third president, Thomas Jefferson, wore his own hair throughout his life parted simply and falling to just below the shoulder**

the shoulder, and with a fringe (fig. 61). As emperor, he changed his hairstyle yet again. To look like a king was not good enough for him. It was also quite contrary to the whole concept of the revolution. Napoleon looks back instead to an earlier precedent – the Roman Empire. So we see him next in fig. 62 with ears revealed and short hair brushed forward across the brow, every inch the Roman emperor.

Meanwhile, back in the lady's boudoir, the change

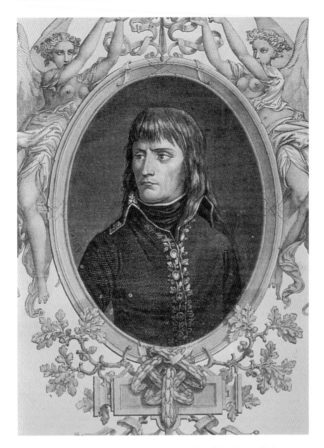

FIG. 61. Young Napoleon — shoulder-length hair with a fringe.
Portrait of Napoleon Bonaparte, engraved by Stephane Pannemaker after Eugène Josephe Viollat, nineteenth century (private collection)

young English girl in fig. 65. She, in common with her far more sophisticated French counterpart, wears the 'empire line' with its distinctive high waist just below her breasts – the Titus cut and the empire line, indeed, seem almost inseparable. Her shaggy short cut has something of the shaggy mane of the pony that stands beside her. So it is that the picture also illustrates so well, athough incidentally, a small girl's ageless and universal desire to identify herself with her favourite pet. Indeed, were she wearing jodphurs, she could be the quintessential pony club member of today.

More in Madame Recamier's league, in England, was Mary Anne Clarke. She was, indeed, close to being

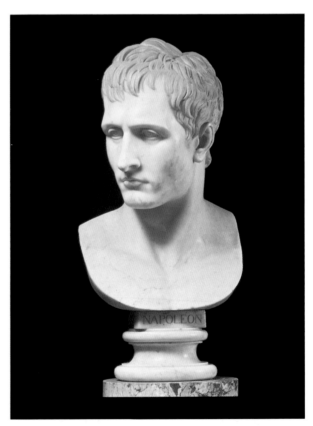

FIG. 62. Napoleon the Emperor — short-haired like a Roman senator.
Antonio Canova, marble portrait bust of Napoleon Bonaparte, nineteenth century
(Galleria d'Arte Moderna, Florence)

was no less dramatic – indeed it was more so, because, rather than follow classical female styles to complement their emperor's Roman revival, the more daring females copied Napoleon himself and had their hair cut short. They did not call the style 'a Napoleon' but described it, rather less blatantly, as *à la Titus*. It recalled that Roman 'pin-up' from the third century, Titus, the son of Vespasian. That leader both of fashion and thought, Madame Recamier, is seen in fig. 63 with her hair – and a fair abundance of it – bound *à la Grecque* some time around 1798–9. By 1800, in David's famous portrait of her (fig. 64), it is much shorter, but not yet quite as severe as the true Titus, worn rather surprisingly by the

Madame Recamier's English counterpart. Mistress to the Duke of York, she was bribed to obtain army promotions and eventually imprisoned for libel, ending her days in Paris. Figs 66 and 67 show her transition from the long-haired to the short. The latter also shows a willingness to reveal a nipple in the cause of art, seen rather more dramatically in what is perhaps the most vivid picture of the Titus style (fig. 68). The unknown girl, rather than wearing an empire line dress with the high waist pressing up beneath her breasts, goes a stage further than Mary Anne Clarke and has both of them bare. She clasps them in a manner that is both provocative and self-indulgent. The psychologist might claim that, having lost her long hair, she feels the need to protect her body instead with her hands. Or, again, no longer able to run her fingers through her tresses, she seeks alternative comfort by feeling her breasts. Whatever you read into it, this is an extraordinarily powerful picture that could easily have been painted not in 1812 but some time after the bra-burning, hair-cutting, post-Female Eunuch part of the twentieth century.

However, it was not just Napoleon and conscious imitation of Greece and Rome that motivated the changes in styles, but the social necessity of distancing oneself from the *ancien régime*. Just as men were wearing trousers rather than breeches to assimilate themselves with the *sans culottes*, so women were setting aside the elaborate hairstyles that had literally fallen under the guillotine, just as Charles I's had under the axe.

From those dynamic short-haired women, it is perhaps a relief to turn to a long-haired beauty. Like them, Emma Hamilton (fig. 69) wears the empire line. For the artist, representing his sitter as a bacchante is an excuse for letting her hair down with some degree of propriety. The picture shows us why so many men loved Lady Hamilton – the painter of this portrait, George Romney, not least among them. *The Dictionary of National Biography* records that, in 1782 (surely the year in which this picture was painted?), she was 'refined by innocent intimacy with him'. Less innocent were her other encounters, particularly that with Nelson, with whom she became intimate in 1798, the relationship lasting until his death as a hero at Trafalgar. However,

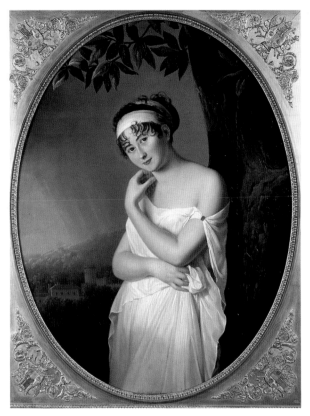

FIG. 63. Hair à la Grecque – the first step towards the short or 'Titus' look.
Eulalie Morin, *Portrait of Madame Recamier,*
1800 (Chateau de Versailles)

the well-known portrait of her that was hanging in the great cabin of HMS Victory on that fateful day is that of a very demure-looking woman bearing a startling resemblance to the short-haired Madame Recamier, her contemporary in enemy France.

However, if Nelson's treasured picture of her shows her with short hair, another picture of the period (fig. 70) poses a puzzle. Painted little more than two years before Trafalgar, it shows her with tresses that are, if anything, even more voluminous than those to be seen in fig. 69.

However, it seems that we should not believe all the artist shows us or the lady would have us think. For all is revealed when one turns to the journal of Mrs M. St George. Writing about breakfasting with Lady Hamilton

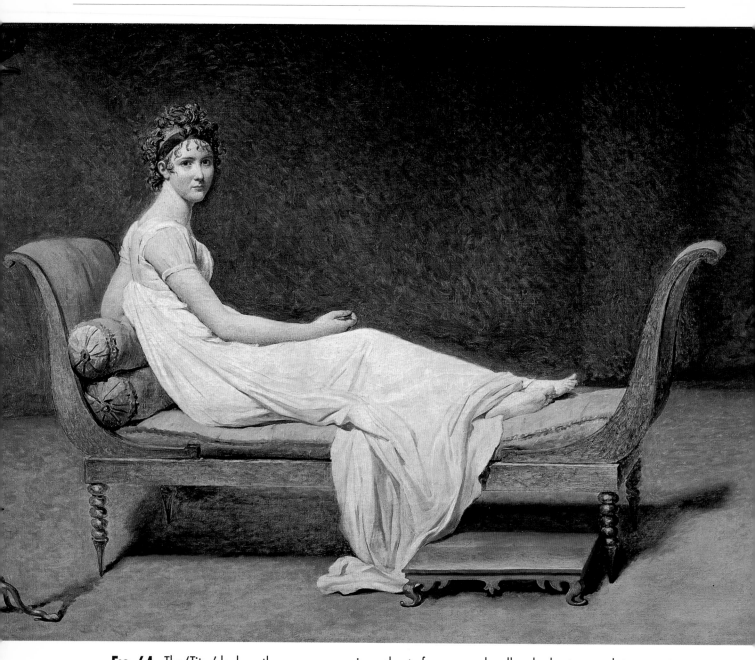

FIG. 64. The 'Titus' look on the same woman, in moderate form over a headband, about a year later.
Jacques Louis David, *Madame Recamier*, 1800
(Louvre Museum, Paris)

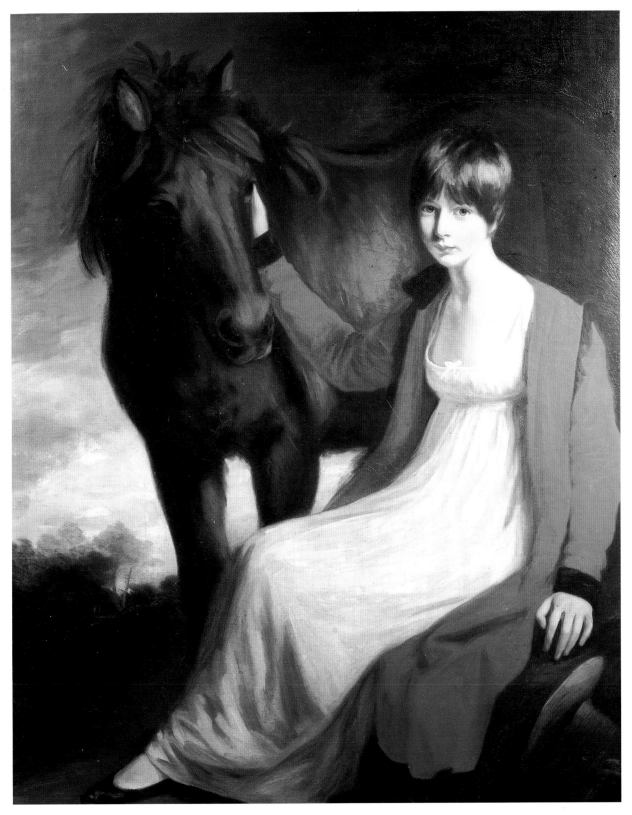

FIG. 65. The true 'Titus' in less sophisticated form.

John Opie, *Miss Emily Beauchamp with her Pony*, eighteenth century (private collection)

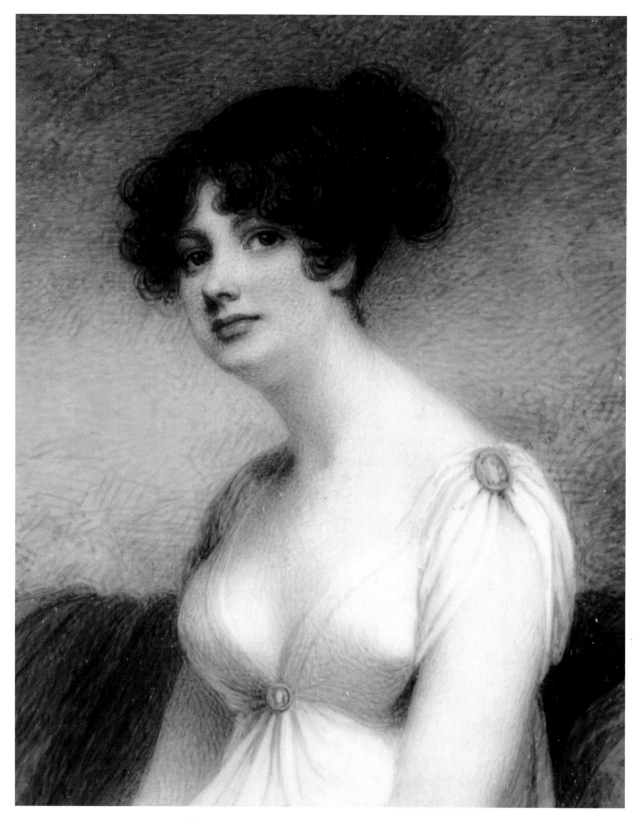

FIG. 66. Long-haired beauty — in the year she became mistress to the Duke of York.
Adam Buck, *Mary Anne Clarke* (miniature), 1803 (National Portrait Gallery, London)

While Emma, Lady Hamilton had her hair shorn, that of her hero, Lord Nelson, remained long – an unusual and early instance of the male partner's hair being longer than the female's

on 7 October 1800, she observes that 'her hair (which by the bye is never clean) is short, dressed like an antique'. In other words, clean or dirty, Lady Hamilton's hair was cut *à la Grecque*, if not as short as the Titus cut, in 1800 or before. She certainly would not have had time to grow it again to the extreme length seen in fig. 70 in the space of just three years. The solution is, of course, simple. She must surely have retained the hair she had shed for use in striking her classical poses, the 'attitudes' for which she was famous. Indeed, on looking at her temples it becomes clear that the hair which is actually growing on her head is really quite short and curly. The red headband must surely have had sewn to it the hair that had been shorn in the cause of fashion, only to be worn again, briefly, in the cause of art – her own hair, certainly, but only in a manner of speaking.

While Emma, Lady Hamilton had her hair shorn, that of her hero, Lord Nelson, remained long – an unusual and early instance of the male partner's hair being longer than the female's. Fig. 71 shows Lord Nelson's pigtail hanging down his back, bound from nape to tip in ribbon. It is not a contemporary record – one does not normally record a hero's back view – but a faithful reconstruction at Madame Tussaud's. Nelson's hair is naturally grey, which is as well, since Pitt's government required anyone powdering their hair to acquire a licence to do so at the price of one guinea a year. The so-called 'guinea-pigs' paid £210,136 in total in that first year. Not surprisingly, the fashion came to an end shortly afterwards. Nelson, as a sailor, did not wear a wig since it would obviously have been embarrassing were it to be blown overboard. For equally

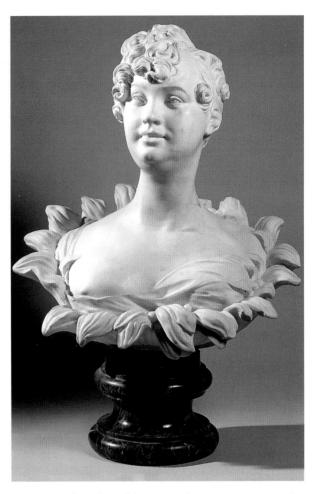

FIG. 67. Short-haired beauty – the same woman eight years later, with her 'Titus' haircut.
Lawrence Gahagan, small marble bust of Mary Anne Clarke, 1811 (National Portrait Gallery, London)

practical reasons sailors, from the highest to the lowest, wore their hair long, simply binding it further as it grew. By the time of Trafalgar, however, Nelson's military equivalent, Wellington, had hair quite as short as their common adversary, Napoleon.

In the American army, 1 April 1801 was a remarkable day, for it was then that General Wilkinson ordered that the hair of all soldiers should be 'cropped, without exception of persons'. In the event there was one exception, Lieutenant Colonel Thomas Butler, who defiantly retained his long hair. He was given special dispensation on 2

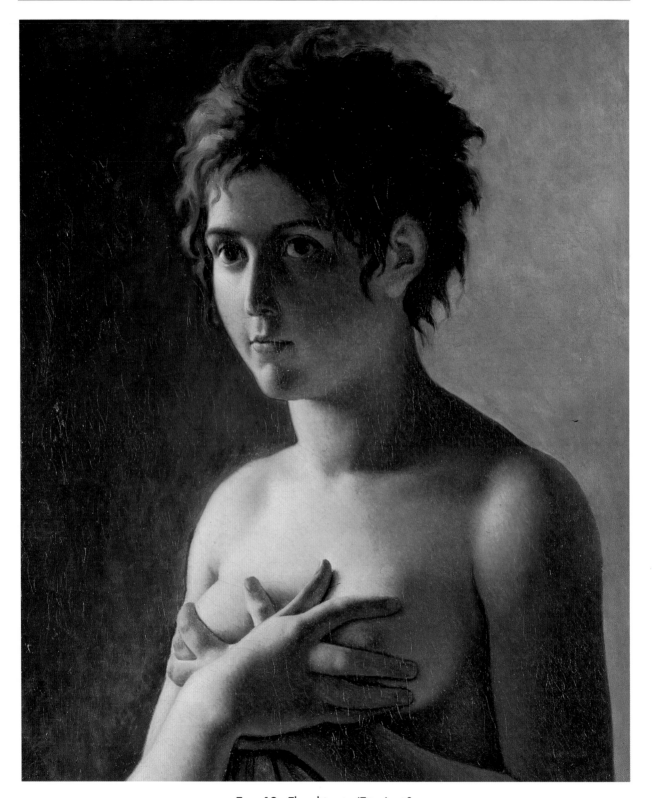

FIG. 68. The ultimate 'Titus' cut?
Baron Pierre-Narcisse Guérin,
Portrait of a Young Girl, 1812 (Louvre Museum, Paris)

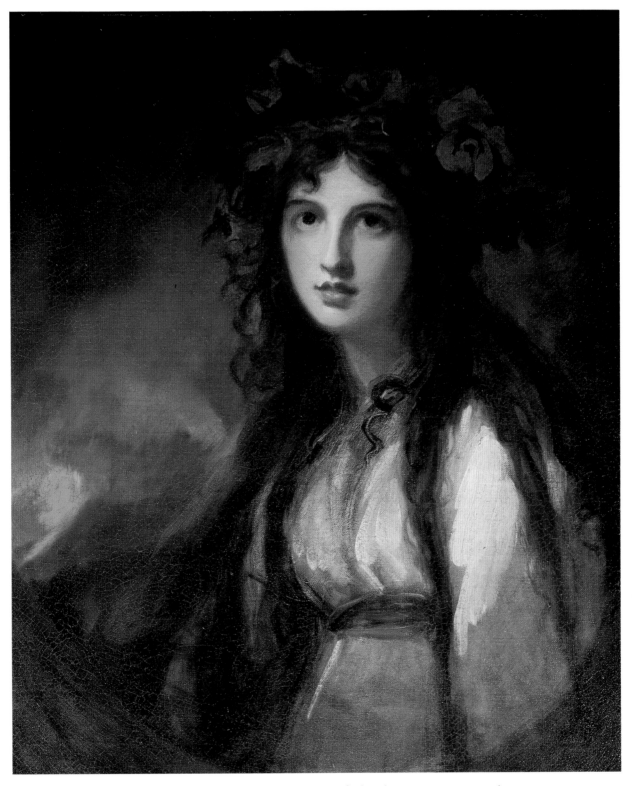

FIG. 69. Simple long-haired beauty personified – the young Emma Hamilton.
George Romney, *Portrait of Emma, Lady Hamilton* (c.1765–1815)
(Philip Mould Historical Portraits Ltd, London)

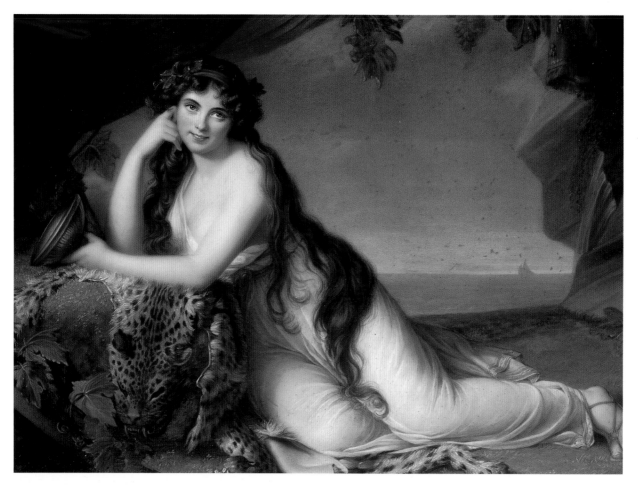

FIG. 70. Long or short? — the apparently long-haired Emma Hamilton as she posed for the artist two years before the Battle of Trafalgar, with abundant locks, despite reports in 1800 that her hair had been cut short. Henry Bone, *Lady Hamilton as a Bacchante*, c.1803 (Wallace Collection, London)

August, when General Wilkinson ordered that he could 'in consideration of his infirm health' continue to wear his hair long. There are plenty of instances where hair has been cut in the interest of good health, but seldom has it been retained on medical grounds, so this face-saving formula hardly has the ring of credibility.

Where the American army led, the British army followed. There came another remarkable day, this time in 1808, when the entire British army paraded, regiment upon regiment. When the order was given, every soldier turned and smartly cut off the pigtail of the soldier in front of him. The entire operation, we are told, was completed in ten minutes. Only a few years before,

soldiers whose hair was not of adequate length were required to wear wigs or false pigtails to conform with those soldiers with naturally long hair. Changing times!

George III had caused dismay among wig makers when he ascended the throne in 1760 wearing not a wig but his own hair. The fashion for wigs, introduced by a Scottish king of England from France, Charles II, was now to go into decline as this third, but first English-born, Hanoverian king started his long reign. In vain did the wig makers of London appeal to him, in 1765, to require every adult citizen, by law, to wear a wig. However, George III's part in the downfall of the wig was a subtle one, because in fact he dressed his hair to

So, during this remarkable time George III assisted in the disappearance of the wig, and Napoleon, in turn, led the way to the shortening of a man's natural hair. However, more dramatically still, Madame Recamier and her like, on both sides of the Channel, willingly cut their long tresses. Would heads ever appear quite the same again?

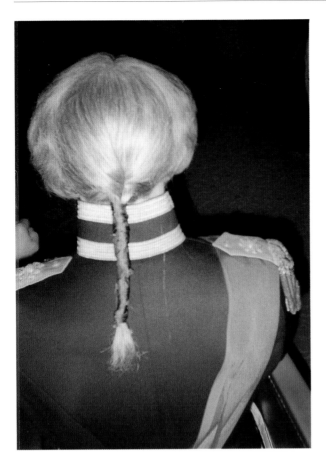

FIG. 71. Horatio Nelson's hair was longer than Emma Hamilton's. Nelson's pigtail is recreated in a modern waxwork at Madame Tussaud's (photo author)

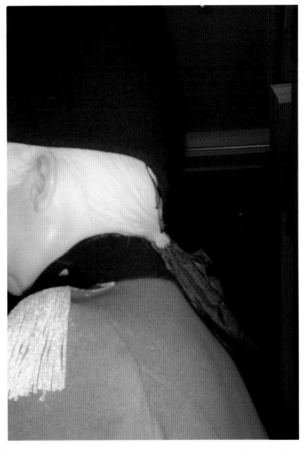

FIG. 72. George III kept his hair in a little bag at the back of his neck in order to keep the powder off his clothes, as if it were a 'bag-wig', tied with a bow at the front of his neck (the origin of today's bow tie). George III's hair disguised to look like a bag-wig, modern waxwork at Madame Tussaud's (photo author)

look as much like a wig as possible, wearing it as if it were a 'bag wig'. The essential elements of this are not readily seen in any contemporary portrait, since (as with Nelson) a great man is usually shown from the front rather than the back. However, again Madame Tussaud assists us (fig. 72). His queue or pigtail is contained within a little black satin bag, designed to keep the powder off his jacket. This bag is secured with ribbons around the neck that are tied at the front, beneath the chin, in a neat bow. This is the origin of the formal bow tie that men wear today. How many realise that, in doing so, they would have you believe that they have a pigtail hanging down their back in a bag? It is certainly evidence that it is not just female fashion that can be nonsensical.

CROWNING GLORY:

PLAIN OR RINGLETS WITH A BUN

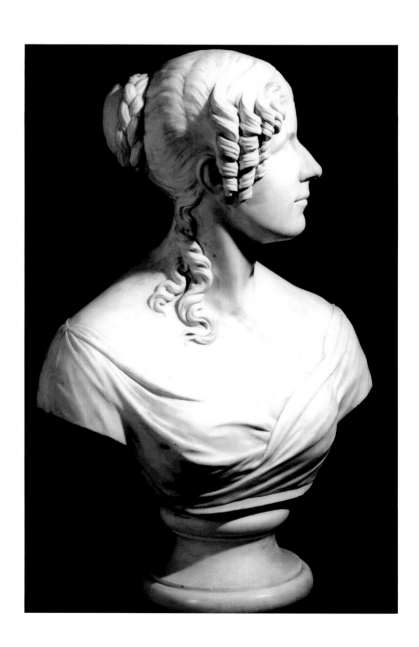

FIG. 73. The precursor of hairstyles of
the Victorian age — three ringlets in
front of the ear and
a bun behind the head.
Angus Fletcher, plaster bust of Felicia
Dorothea Hemans, 1829 (National
Portrait Gallery, London)

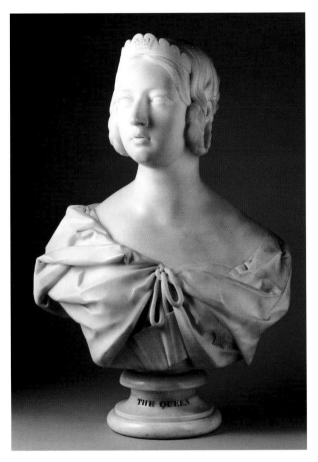

FIG. 74. The young Queen Victoria wearing her hair *à la Clothilde*.
Sir Francis Chantrey, marble bust of Queen Victoria, c.1839
(National Portrait Gallery, London)

Queen Victoria was central to the nineteenth century from girlhood to old age. Her hairstyle was to be as influential, throughout her empire and beyond, as that of Napoleon was throughout his. Numismatists still refer to the 'bun penny', the penny upon which the young Victoria is seen in profile, with her hair in a 'bun' at the back of her head. Surtees, who ranks with Trollope, Thackeray and Dickens as an observer of nineteenth-century society, called one of his novels *Plain or Ringlets?* The title echoes a Victorian girl's agonising decision, as she sits before her mirror, as to whether she should wear her hair straight or curled.

It also echoes the young man's quandary as to which he prefers in the female of his dreams. The hair of a girl, be she queen or commoner, was universally revered as her 'crowning glory', an essentially Victorian sentiment which, in the realm of the girl-queen, made every girl a queen. Her hair was to be treasured, seldom or never to be cut, always to be carefully tended and only to be let down in private.

However, it is to an Italian rather than Victoria that we turn first – Antonio Canova. He carved *The Three*

> **The hair of a girl, be she queen or commoner, was universally revered as her 'crowning glory'**

Graces initially for Napoleon's estranged empress, Josephine, but when she proved backward in coming forward with the deposit, the Duke of Bedford took over the commission. So it was that this superb sculpture was installed in a special temple at Woburn Abbey in 1819. In 1795 there had been something of a revolution in the wearing of hair when the Duke of Bedford and his friends solemnly cut off their pigtails one day at Woburn, rather than contribute to Pitt's tax on powder for hair. Canova himself must have influenced the fashion of shorter hair for men with his bust of Napoleon in true Roman senatorial style (fig. 62). Fifteen years later his incomparable *Three Graces* must, likewise, have assisted in setting a style, this time – for women at least – restoring the popularity of long hair. That, anyway, is my theory. All three are certainly well endowed with luxuriant locks and are so well known, to this day, as not to require further reproduction.

The Empress Josephine enthused about Canova's concept of depicting the Three Graces, assuming that it was an original idea of his. He did not contradict her, but there was, of course, ample classical precedent for

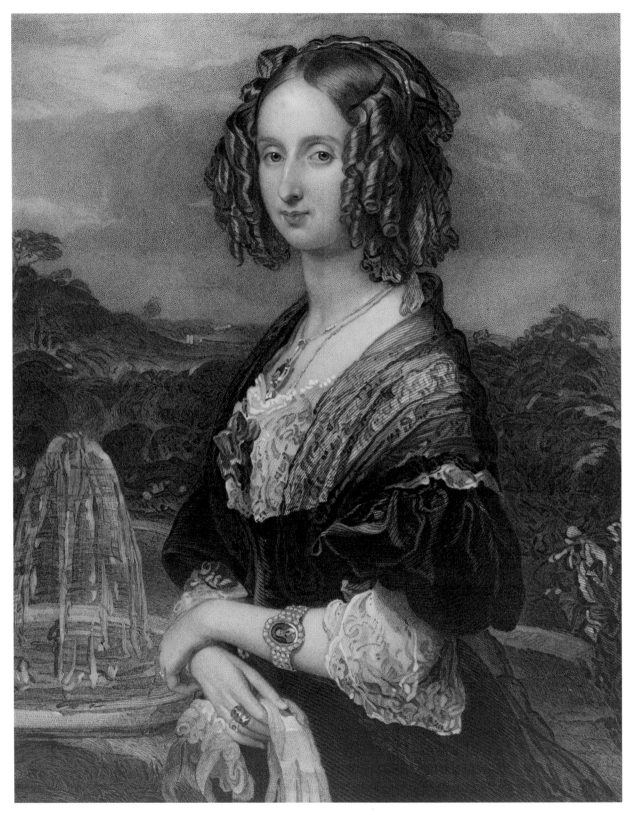

FIG. 75. Ringlets in profusion. *Queen Louisa of the Belgians,* H. Robinson after Sir William C. Ross RA (author's collection)

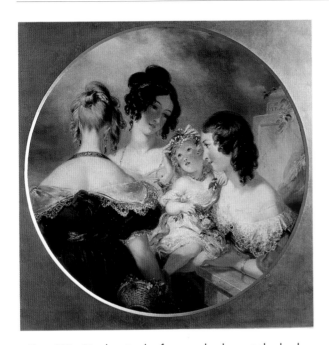

FIG. 76. Ringlets in the front and a bun at the back could result in a rather strange rear view.
Edmund Thomas Parris, *The Lily*
(Victoria & Albert Museum, London)

such a concept. It was simply a matter of moving rather further back from the Titus cut to the abundant and intricate tresses of the Greek goddess. Canova's *Three Graces*, standing in their temple at Woburn, must surely have had their influence on all who saw them. While gentlemen would have admired their bottoms, able to view them unabashed since this was 'art', the ladies could wonder at the intricacy of their hairstyles. But how could one translate a virtuoso performance by a sculptor in that hard but, once carved, finite material of marble into a transient arrangement of one's own hair at the hands of a hairdresser?

Nine years after *The Three Graces* arrived at Woburn, and eight years before Queen Victoria ascended the throne, one very personable and beautiful lady wore a hairstyle that combined the elegance of *The Three Graces* with the propriety and reasonable practicality of the Victorian age that lay ahead. That lady was Felicia Dorothea Hemans. In fig. 73 she wears her front hair in three ringlets from the temple down to the lobe of

her ear, which nestles behind them. At the nape of her neck, two locks of hair hang freely to her shoulder. Finally, she has the remainder of her back hair plaited at its base and wound around a bun formed of the upper part. Here, then, is a bun, ringlets and plain hair. Felicia Dorothea Hemans was a poet, seen here in her mid-thirties, when she was a close friend of both Wordsworth and Scott. Her writings were highly popular in America, as, one feels sure, she herself would have been had she ever set foot there. To borrow a phrase coined in the 1970s to describe a television arts correspondent, Joan Bakewell, she must surely rank as being 'the thinking man's crumpet'.

Victoria was just nineteen years old and one year into her reign when Sir Francis Chantrey made his preliminary sketches for her bust (fig. 74). The finished article looks very composed, complete with diadem. If you go to the National Portrait Gallery you will see that the sketches, full face and side view, reveal the queen as the child she was. Her forehair is parted to a point level with the ears, fore and aft. The back hair, separated by the ear-to-ear parting, is plaited and wound into a bun, with the two plaits of the forehair brought up to join it, looping under each ear. The style is similar to that worn by Felicia Dorothea Hemans but with the

Obviously, the young queen's hairstyle was to have a very profound effect upon those of her young contemporaries

plaits taking the place of ringlets, which would have needed to be a lot shorter than was practical with Victoria's full head of hair. The result, certainly in sketch form as opposed to the finished bust, is to create the effect of a child hardly out of nursery, only with her plaits looped up rather than hanging loose. Obviously, the young queen's hairstyle was to have a very profound

The simpler hairstyle of the girl in profile shows the neck and ears covered in a fashion that is rather more attractive to modern eyes

effect upon those of her young contemporaries. Every mother, at least, would wish her daughter to emulate her. The style might almost be called *à la Victoria*. In fact, it was called *à la Clothilde* and was not limited to the English or the young.

The serious little queen would not wish, or could not be allowed, to indulge in extremes of fashion. Louisa, the young French born Queen of the Belgians would seem to have no such qualms (fig. 75). If you were a ringlets man she would be your 'Pin-Up' – literally so since she appears here as the frontispiece in the *Keepsake* Annual of 1844. The girl with her back to us in fig. 76 reveals a somewhat starkly naked nape, contrasting with her side hair dangling on either side of her bare ears. The girl she faces must look equally strange from behind. Juvenal would surely have found it quite as amusing, as he did the rear view of the orbis hairstyle of his own time (fig. 17). The simpler hairstyle of the girl in profile shows the neck and ears covered in a fashion that is rather more attractive to modern eyes.

There is nothing to beat the portrait of a woman leaning forward over her work to highlight a hairstyle. As with Vermeer's lacemaker two centuries before (fig. 47), so with William Etty's crochet worker (fig. 77), The crochet worker, Miss Mary Anne Purdon, has her hair parted simply in the centre. It is then swept to either side in soft folds over her ears to join the bun at the back of her head, her back hair having been parted from side to side very close to the crown. One can imagine her arranging it herself unaided. She is clearly handy with her crochet hooks, so why not with her hairpins?

Indeed, she could almost be the same girl as depicted in fig. 78, who holds one part of her hair up while the rest falls free. This is the tricky moment in which one hand keeps the hair in place, while the other brings the remaining hair up to join it. It is the sort of moment that a man would like to chance upon, either in the flesh or aided and abetted, as here, by the artist. One side of the hair up in civilised form and the other hanging down in wild abandon is (or was) the sort of contrast that sets the male heart fluttering.

The contrast is better still if the girl, seemingly unaware of her audience, is unselfconsciously naked, as is the charming Danish woman standing in front of a mirror (fig. 79). Painted in 1841, she is surely almost the direct contemporary of the young Queen Victoria, but her simpler hairstyle is almost identical to that of the girls in figs 77 and 78. A moment before, her hair would have been covering her now naked back or falling forwards over the naked breast which one sees in the mirror. She stands looking at her pin box, as if deciding which pins to dive into the hair that she holds ready in a bun. The mirror shows clearly her T-shaped partings: from the neck upwards she looks ready for the drawing room. From the neck downwards she looks quite the reverse. Little did she know that her form was to adorn hoardings all over London advertising Jonathan Miller's 1998 exhibition at the National Gallery on the theme of 'Reflections'. Of all the thousands who saw her, one wonders how many noticed, as she clearly has yet to notice, a teasing irregularity. Whereas her hair (so we see in the mirror) loops softly over her right ear, totally hiding it, her left ear stands out looking rather pink and ugly. This is because the hair on her left side has been drawn severely back behind it, leaving it standing proud. Poor girl! Once she has securely pinned the hair and

Fig. 77. A simpler style with hair swept over the ears to a bun at the back.
William Etty, *Study for the crochet worker, Miss Mary Anne Purdon* (York City Art Gallery)

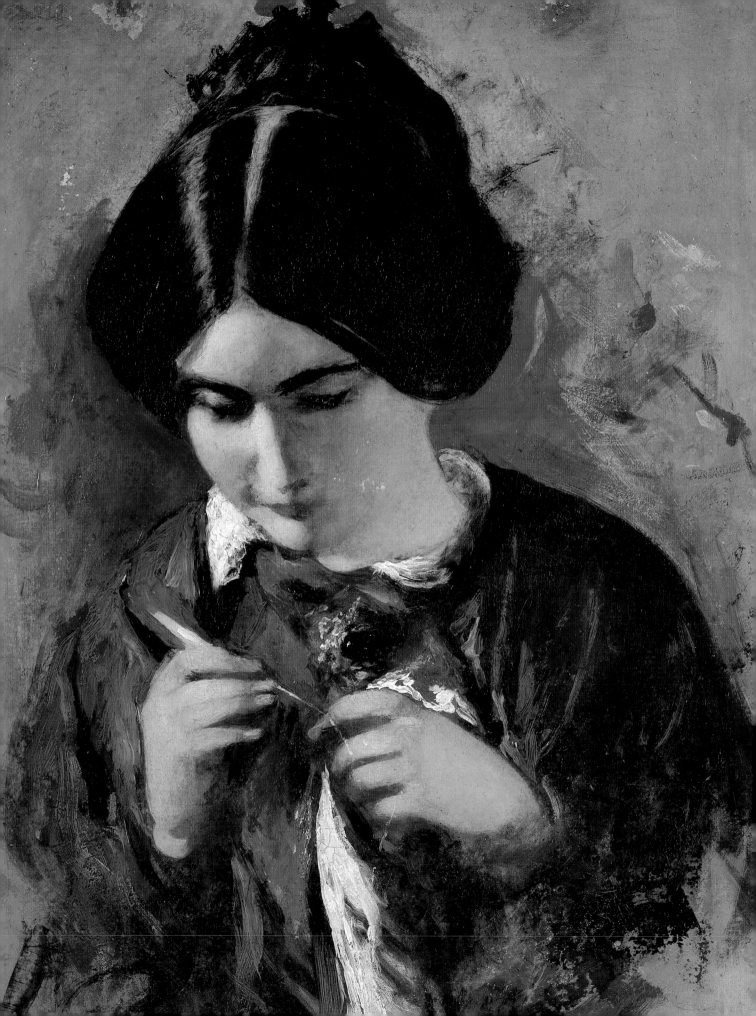

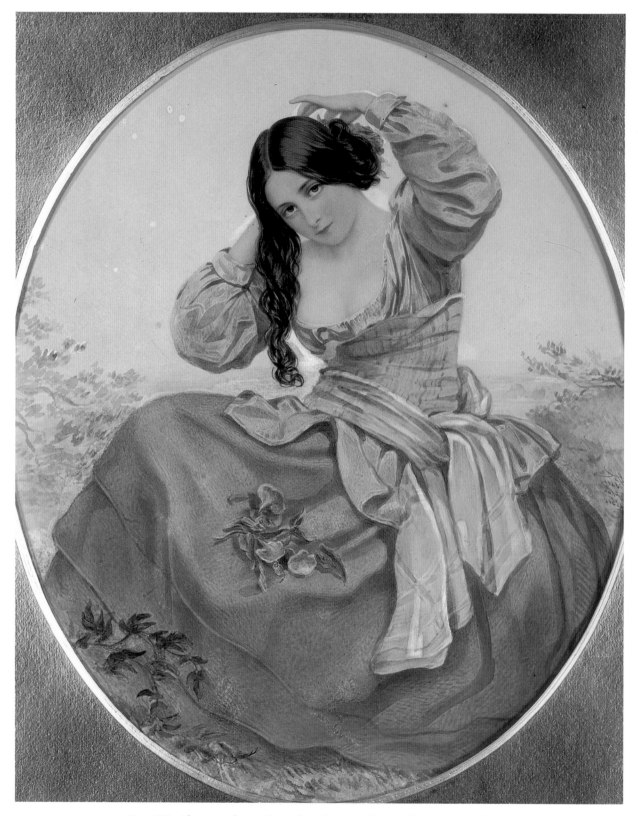

FIG. 78. The same hairstyle as that shown in fig. 78, being put in place.
James Fisher, *A Rustic Toilet* (Maidstone Museum and Art Gallery, Kent)

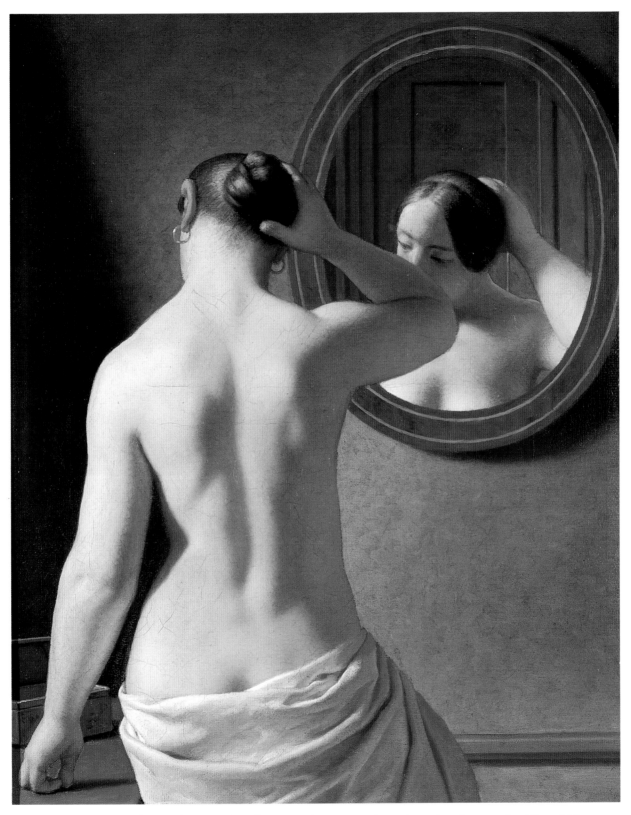

FIG. 79. A bun about to be pinned in place, completing a similar style to that shown in figs 78 and 79.
Christoffer Wilhelm Eckersberg, *Woman Standing in Front of a Mirror*, 1841

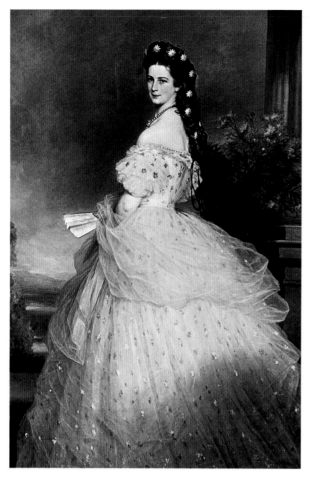

FIG. 80. Long hair worn loose but adorned
with rosettes.
Franz Xavier Winterhalter ,
Elizabeth, Empress of Austria (private collection)

looked at herself full face in the mirror, she will realise her mistake and have to start all over again.

It would not have been surprising, then, if a girl were to grow tired of her long hair. That is, unless she had someone to tend it for her. Luckily, behind most elegantly coiffured ladies was a lady's maid who would take infinite care in dressing her mistress's hair. Even if a society lady left her hair down it needed constant brushing, and this too would normally have been done by her maid (although she could of course have performed the task herself, particularly if she leant forward and brushed her hair in front of her face rather than attempting to do it behind her own back).

It is doubtful that Elizabeth of Bavaria would have brushed her own hair. Understandably proud of her fine, flowing mane, she continued to wear it loose rather than putting it up even when she became Empress of Austria, no doubt to the delight of her courtiers. In the portrait of her reproduced here (fig. 80) – lest people should think she had wandered into a ballroom without taking the trouble to have her hair dressed, perhaps – her long hair is studded with star-like rosettes. They sit like a coronet around her head and trail like a dazzling torrent of stars down her back. Propriety, though, would have required that lesser mortals view her thus only within the safe confines of a picture frame.

Certainly in polite English society, long flowing hair was generally acceptable only in girlhood, whereas a widow, however young, was expected to wear hers not only up but also covered. So it is that the veiled Queen Victoria in fig. 81 plays the part of age, gazing wistfully at the youthful flowing hair of her daughter Beatrice. The child is hardly younger than she was herself at the beginning of her reign. The Queen, widowed before her time, has an open book on her lap, symbolic perhaps of a new chapter.

Down or up, visible or covered, long hair was back to stay throughout Victoria's reign and would remain so, with very few exceptions, until the scissors came out again at the end of the First World War.

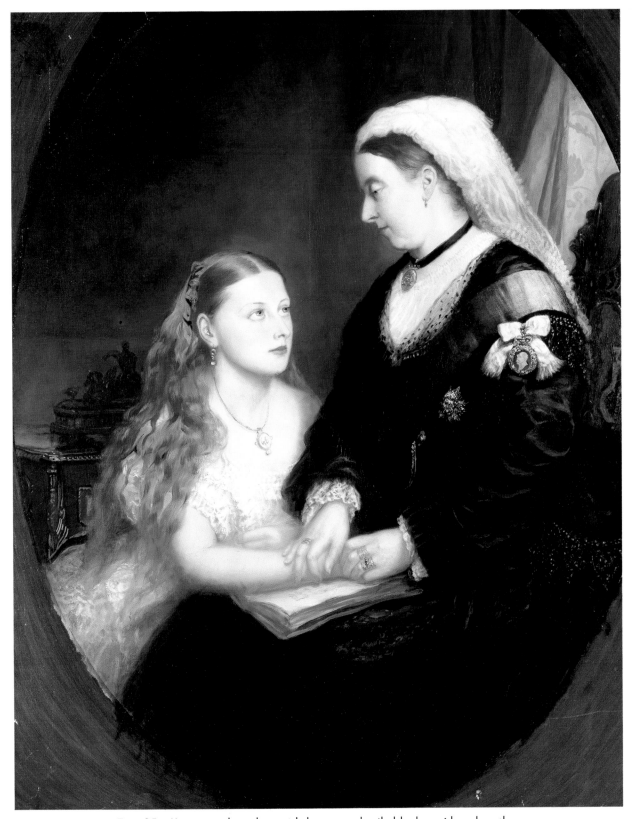

FIG. 81. Hair worn down by a girl, but up and veiled by her widowed mother.
Unknown artist, *Princess Beatrice and Queen Victoria* (National Portrait Gallery, London)

LA VIE PARISIENNE

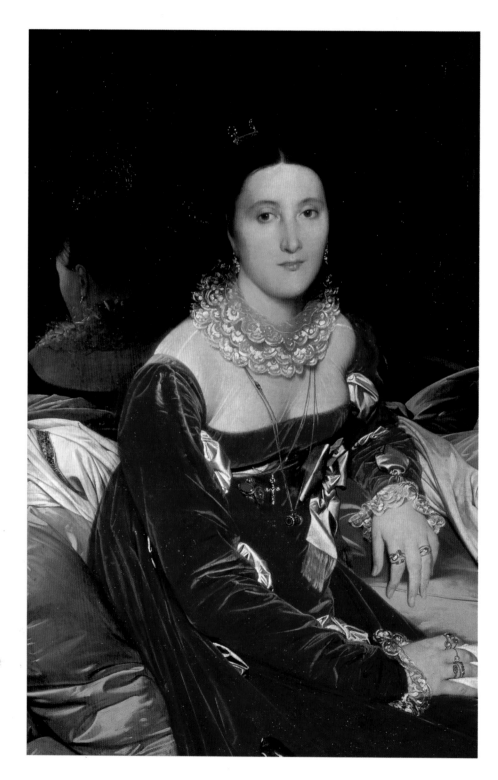

FIG. 82. The hair as a dark frame for the face. Jean Auguste Dominique Ingres, *Madame de Senonnes* (Musée des Beaux-Arts, Nantes)

While hair might have been predominantly long throughout Europe, there was a world of difference between the style in which it was worn in Victorian England, or at the courts of Victoria's various cousins, and that to be found in the capital of France's Second Empire. In Paris hair, clothes and décolletage – offering those tantalising glimpses of skin – became fused into one great stylish trinity, no one element subordinate to the other. The ensemble was everything, and capturing it in a salon painting for society's admiration and approval was the summit of a lady's ambition.

The Impressionists' subjects come across not as Barbie dolls but as real flesh, blood and hair

Many portrait painters were bossed about by their sitters, who looked upon them as no more than the equivalent of today's commercial photographer. Not so Ingres, who often dictated not only what his subject wore but also how she should dress her hair. In his portrait of Madame de Senonnes (fig. 82) he uses the hair to set the face in sharp relief, rather than as a feature in itself. It is the flesh of the parting, rather than the hair on either side, which is of importance, looking like the stem of a pear leading the eye up from her oval face. The hair, drawn back into a bun behind the head, disappears into obscurity, the jewels set in it being more important than the hair itself. Again, although Ingres positions his sitter in front of a mirror, this is to draw our eye not to the hair at the back of her head but, rather, to the bare nape of her neck and her shapely uncovered ear with its jewelled pendant.

After such sophisticated restraint, it is a relief to come to the relatively innocent freshness of the Impressionists in general and Renoir in particular as we enter the last quarter of the nineteenth century. The salon painters, such as Ingres, part recorded and part created fashion. The Impressionists, at first voluntarily banishing themselves to the *Salon des refusés*, naturally also had to have an eye to their patrons' aspirations. However, at the same time they could show them and their children as real people, using a natural approach contrasting with the artificiality of the dolls that were still used to convey hair and clothing designs around the world. The Impressionsists' subjects come across not as Barbie dolls but as real flesh, blood and hair. The girl we met in fig. 4 must speak for all of them, though it would be tempting to fill this whole chapter with images of Renoir's young girls with hair up, hair down, at the piano, in their pinafores or in their Sunday best.

But we must move on to a lesser artist and a less innocent age, for the 'Parisienne' style is also about coquettish temptation. Indeed, fig. 83 is entitled *The Coquette*. In it we see the back of the head. We also see the girl's naked nape, and we are reminded that the nape of the neck is one of the most sensitive of the

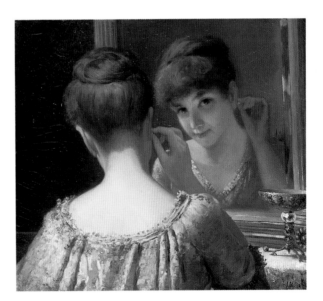

FIG. 83. Coquettish charm – the girl's reflected eye looks not at herself but captivatingly across her shoulder at the intimate observer.
James Wells Champney, *The Coquette* (c.1885)
(private collection/Christie's Images)

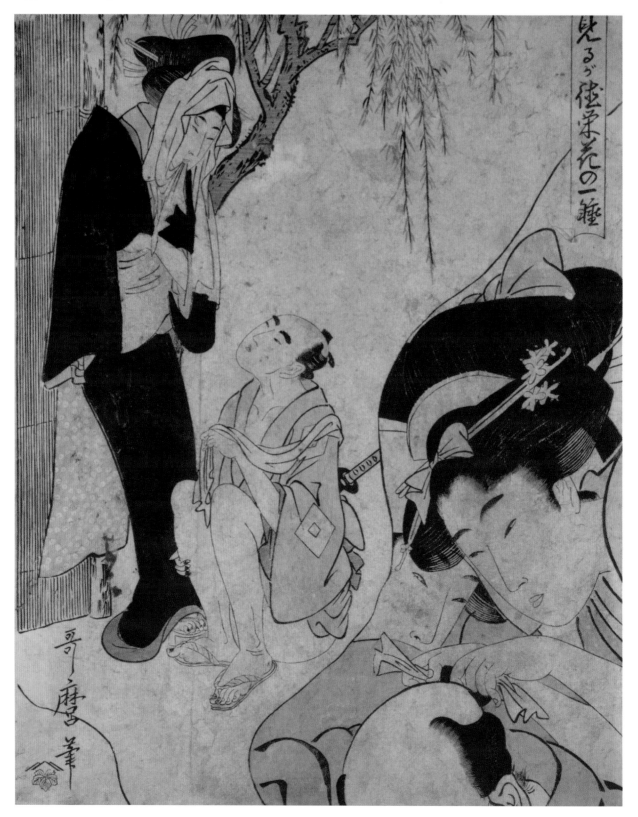

見るゝ徒栄花の一種

FIG. 84. Japanese hairstyles inspired Western imitation.

A nineteenth-century Japanese woodblock (Dodge and Sons, Sherborne)

Parisian society borrowed from other cultures as and when it suited, as much in hairstyles as in style of clothing

erogenous zones. The painter seems to invite the viewer to bend down and kiss it. The girl's ears, too, are exposed, likewise waiting to be brushed by some Parisian moustache in an afternoon encounter behind carefully drawn blinds. The girl has her hair twisted into a simple bun perched on the crown of her head, like a little pillbox hat. Surely this is hair put up in expectation of it being deftly allowed to tumble, released by some eager male hand. This is indeed hair seen in the very practical role of an essential weapon in a girl's sexual armoury.

The essence of *la vie parisienne*, whether lived in Paris itself or emulated elsewhere, was not just stylish sensuality but also eclecticism. Parisian society borrowed from other cultures as and when it suited, as much in hairstyles as in style of clothing. The craze for all things Japanese is evidence of this. Fig. 84 shows an example of the type of Japanese print that started it all. Fig. 85 shows the hairstyle translated from a Japanese to a European head, the hair piled high and skewered with long, decorated needles. Here, in hair quite as much as in any other branch of decoration, one culture is borrowing from another but at the same time adding to it. This young lady knows that she could never pass for a Japanese girl, nor would she necessarily wish to do so, but for the moment she revels in the fantasy. Tomorrow she will have another hairstyle – all part of the fun of the transformations that hair can bring.

From Paris, catalogues and fashion plates were now transported worldwide, taking the place of the dolls that had once conveyed styles in hair and clothing to other countries, not least America. However, America did not always follow European fashion. From the American Civil War (1861–5) comes a splendid anecdote concerning a woman who wrote to the newspapers calling herself simply 'Delilah', though confessing to

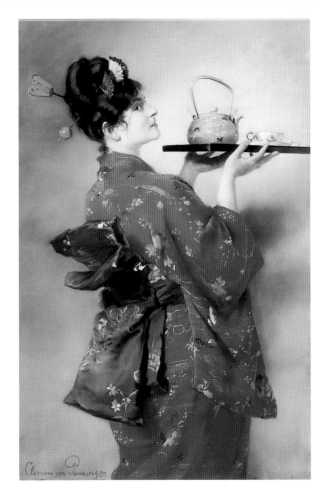

FIG. 85. Black hair piled high and skewered with long needles was the basis of the Japanese style. Clemens von Pausinger, *Portrait of a European lady in Japanese Costume* (John Noott Galleries, Broadway Worcestershire)

being a niece of James Madison. She urged all Confederate women over the age of twelve to cut off their hair and have it transported to Europe. By her reckoning, two million women contributing two braids each, sold at $20 per pair, could go far towards settling the Confederate debt. This tells us a lot about the American woman's propensity for long hair. Had the cry of 'Delilah' been heeded, American heads of hair could have augmented the tresses of the ladies of Paris. However, no such transatlantic traffic is recorded, not at least in support of the Confederate cause.

FIN DE SIÈCLE:

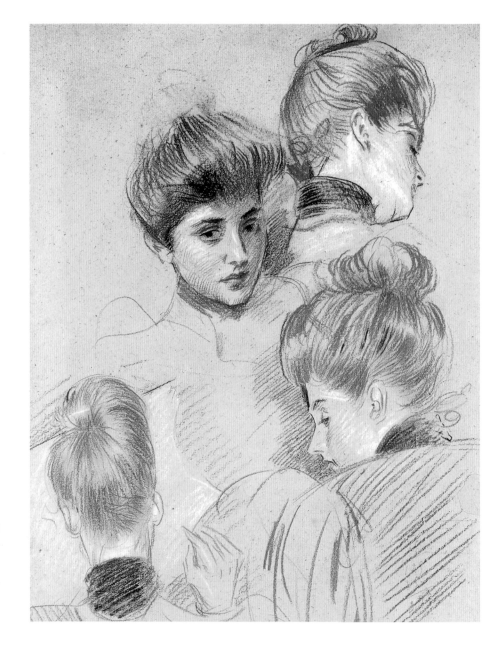

FIG. 86. Soft and curvaceous – Parisian hairstyles at the end of the nineteenth century. Paul César Helleu, *Studies of Mme Helleu and Mme Clarighy,* c.1892–5 (Christopher Wood Gallery, London)

As Victoria's reign ebbed to its close, Parisiènne chic found its way both across the Channel and the Atlantic in a way perhaps not unconnected with her heir's fondness for the ladies of Paris. So it was that the ladies of the Edwardian age, the age which took King Edward's name, were to have a far softer outline to their hair than did their Victorian mothers.

The 'look' and its French origin is epitomised by the studies in fig. 86, which so helpfully show the heads of Madame Helleu and Madame Clarighy from different angles. The sketches emphasise the way in which hair of this period was built up to hang over the brow, rather like the eaves of a thatched cottage. To the right one sees a top knot, no so much like the bun of the early Victorian period as like a cottage loaf. From all angles the emphasis is upon fullness and softness. One finds the same qualities in the American example in fig. 87. Some of these styles could only have been achieved with a discreet insertion of a pad, somewhat unattractively known as a 'rat' to assist the full and rounded effect. This is the chignon - though not, as originally, worn at the nape of the neck, as the word literally implies.

As at the turn of the eighteenth century, so at the turn of the nineteenth, there were those whose hairstyles harked back to the classical, typically with a white head band and a torch-like arrangement of hair rising to a cone. An artist painting such a style might portray his sitter in the guise of 'Daphne' the daughter of a river God, even if in reality she was the daughter of a prosperous London banker.

More interesting than contrived revivals, however, is a glimpse of a very individual family. The painting of the Sitwells (fig. 88) is as fine a record of the hairstyles of its time as is Van Dyck's portrait of Charles I's children (fig. 40). It dates from precisely the turn of the century (1900) and, again like the earlier painting, has a special resonance in that the children in it were all to become well known – in their case, as writers. On the left stands Edith, aged 13, with her medium length hair falling forward over her breast and her distinctive eyes (even then) peering out from beneath her fringe. Her mother, in the centre, here aged about thirty-two, has a similarly

curvacious hairstyle to that of Madames Helleu and Clarighy, topped with a grand hat. Of the two small boys, Sacheverell (aged 3) still in petticoats, like the youngest boy in the Stuart picture of nearly three hundred years before, has curling hair allowed to cover his ears and fall to the nape of his neck. Osbert, aged 8, by contrast, has his cut clear of his pink ears, as befits a boy in a sailor suit (gone are the days of sailors with pigtails). Lastly their forty-year-old father has equally short hair. He looks every inch the conventional country gentleman – which, as it happens, he was far from being. The most important factor here is that, for the first time

As at the turn of the eighteenth century, so at the turn of the nineteenth, there were those whose hairstyles harked back to the classical, typically with a white head band and a torch-like arrangement of hair rising to a cone

in portraiture, England is being portrayed by an American artist: John Singer Sargent, the Van Dyck of the *Fin de Siècle*. Back in his own country, Sargent could bring a sense of grandeur and expression to portraiture, reflecting the new self-confidence of a nation which, in the century ahead, would begin to eclipse both Paris and London in its influence on international taste. In fig. 89 Mrs Fiske Warren looks at us steadily in the eye, from beneath another example of the voluminous but soft hairstyle of the age. However, what makes the picture

Just as John Singer Sargent brought a new standard of portraiture to America that could rival, indeed surpass, any painter in Europe at the time, so Philip Wilson Steer helped to bring Impressionism to England

special is the way in which her daughter Rachel nestles her head in the curve between her mother's neck and left shoulder. Her hair is identical in colour to her mother's but, rather than being pinned up, it is allowed to fall free onto her own left shoulder. The picture almost seems to present two images of the same person, so similar are the faces, the one with the hair up and the other with it down. One can imagine Mrs Fiske Warren sitting in front of her mirror, preparing to put up her hair and seeing, staring back at her, the mirror image of her daughter, despite the twenty-year age gap between them (she is thirty-two in this picture and Rachel twelve).

Just as John Singer Sargent brought a new standard of portraiture to America that could rival, indeed surpass, any painter in Europe at the time, so Philip Wilson Steer helped to bring Impressionism to England. His painting of the back view of girls and their chaperones Watching the Cowes Regatta (fig. 90) brings to an English shore a feeling for hair that is quite as acute as that of Renoir, if rather more sketchily conveyed. One sees, too, in this little picture, female hair through a range of ages. The girls have their backs to us, the better to show us their hair. Because of the age difference, one feels that they

must be sisters, rather than just friends. On that assumption we see that the youngest, with her linen hat, has fairly short but unruly curls, while her middle sister has auburn hair falling half way down her back from beneath a straw hat. Her eldest sister has still longer hair, red and reaching to the waist of her long skirt. It contrasts with her white blouse and is topped by a little blue hat that matches her skirt. One can envisage this eldest sister being teased by her younger siblings about the colour of her hair. They doubtless call her 'Carrots' but are secretly envious of both her hair's length and thickness. They will be impressed, too, when the time comes – probably soon – for her to wear it up, like the mother and aunt (as they must surely be) on the left of the picture. These older women are shown in profile, so that we can see the way in which their hair is worn high on the back of the neck, so as to tilt their jaunty little hats forwards. Finally, is that ghost-like figure at the right-hand-side the grandmother?

Happily one is now in a period where we can turn to popular photographs as well as paintings to get a glimpse of typical hairstyles.

One such photograph is one of a double image taken for viewing in two dimensions, using a stereoscope. Entitled 'Dressing for the Ball', it shows a young lady, only a little older than the oldest girl in the Wilson Steer picture, helpfully showing us both the side and front of her hair, as she stands before a mirror, her maid attending to a flounce on her dress (fig. 91).

We can turn also to photographs of men of the period but they, like the father in the painting of the Sitwells, had their hair short cut. How different it might have been, had it not been for the disgrace of Oscar Wilde, that personification of the male aesthete, shown in fig. 92 in his hey day in 1882. His relatively long hair would have been viewed with acute suspicion, in the case of

FIG. 87. An example of the softer style from America. Robert Reid, *Reflections*, 1891 (Cooley Gallery, Old Lyme, Connecticut)

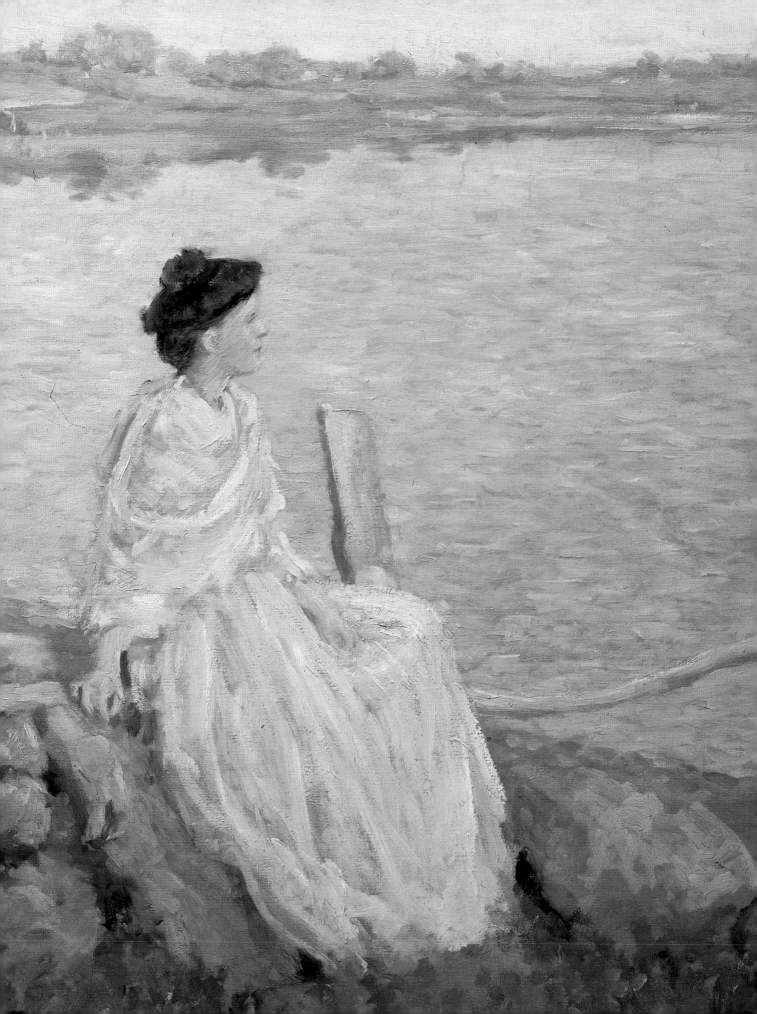

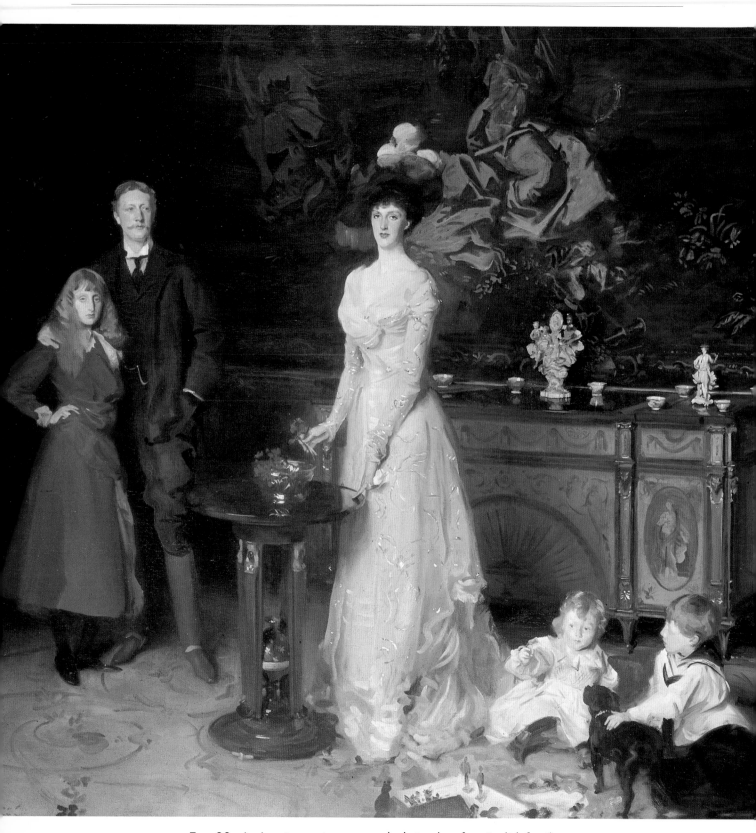

FIG. 88. An American artist captures the hairstyles of an English family.
John Singer Sargent, *The Sitwell Family*, 1900 (private collection)

all but those given special dispensation such as artists, writers and (somewhat surprisingly) the 'Welsh wizard', Lloyd George (fig. 93). However, the exception in the case of Lloyd George is perhaps not surprising. The link between long hair in a man, and homosexuality, was certainly not borne out in the case of this most heterosexual of statesmen. However, even he did not venture to grow his hair longer until relatively old age (the example dates from 1928), being short haired prior to the First World War.

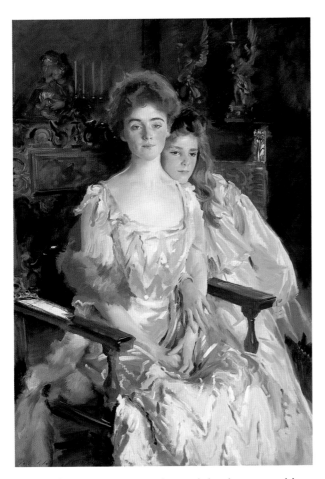

FIG. 89. An American mother with her hair up and her daughter with hers down.
John Singer Sargent, *Mrs Fiske Warren (Gretchen Osgood) and her Daughter Rachel*, 1903 (Museum of Fine Arts, Boston)

The reverse was the case, in this period, concerning the perception of short-haired women (fig. 94), Modigliani's 'Amazon', of 1909, with her collar and tie, waisted jacket and her black hair apparently cut as short as that of any young male bank clerk certainly caused a stir because it seemed to depict a lesbian, so much so that its subject demanded that it be suppressed because she adopted the style, not for sexual reasons, but simply as a matter of practicality, she being a keen horsewoman.

And this is a pointer to the shorter style to come. Most ladies of this age rode side-saddle, a practical way to ride a horse, but one in which fashion dictated that a riding habit be complemented by a full head of hair beneath a hunting top-hat. The lady seen in fig. 95 is clearly mistress of her horse. Nonetheless, she has to use a hand to check that her hat and hair are still safely in place (side-saddle riding has recently enjoyed a great renaissance, but its largely short-haired devotees must wear false buns beneath their hats and veils if they are to achieve that classic look and be as handicapped as their forebears).

Fashion dictated that a riding habit be complemented by a full head of hair beneath a hunting top-hat

The fact of the matter was that women in this *Fin de Siècle* period were beginning to lead far more active lives. Nonetheless, they were still expected to be fully skirted and retain their 'crowning glories'. An example is my own aunt, seen in fig. 96, skiing as a child both in skirt and pigtails. There was also the growing craze of bicycling (fig. 97) requiring ladies to pursue their sport with (at best) divided skirts, topped by hair, hats and veils. Modigliani's 'Amazon' of 1909 was clearly showing the way.

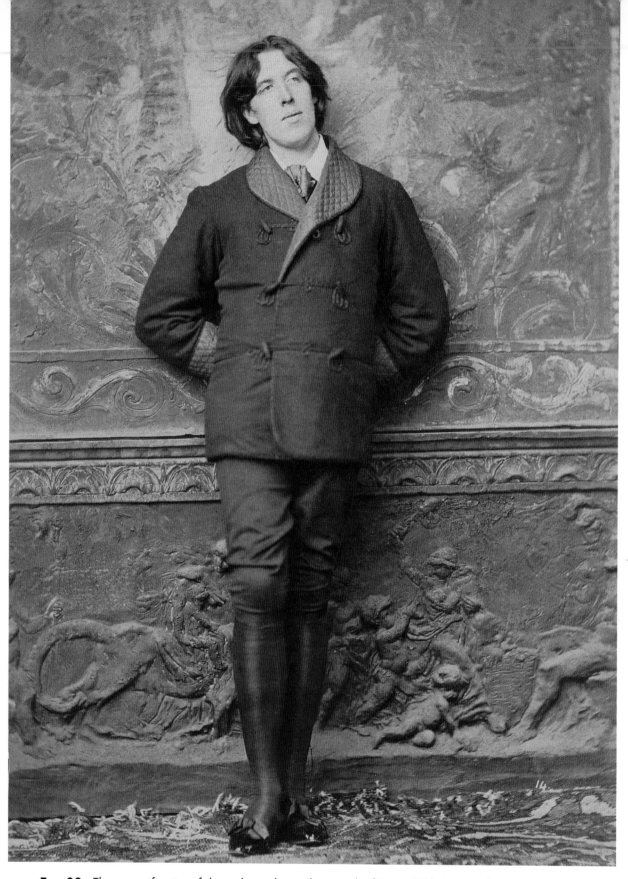

FIG. 92. The personification of the male aesthete. Photograph of Oscar Wilde by Napolean Sarony, 1882 (National Portrait Gallery, London)

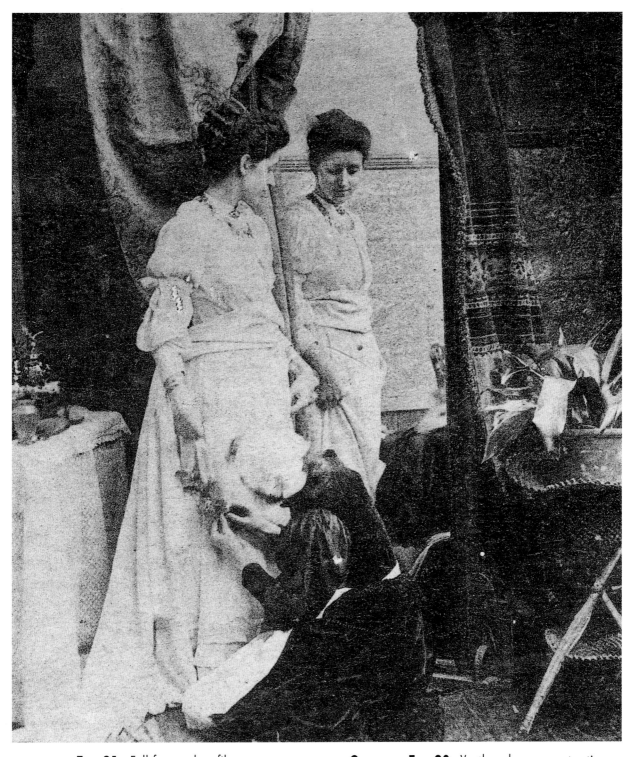

FIG. 91. Full face and profile –
from a contemporary stereoscope
photograph entitled 'Dressing for the Ball'
(author's collection).

OVERLEAF: FIG. 90. Youth and age – contrasting
hairstyles at the seaside.
Philip Wilson Steer, *Watching Cowes Regatta, 1892*
(Southampton City Art Gallery)

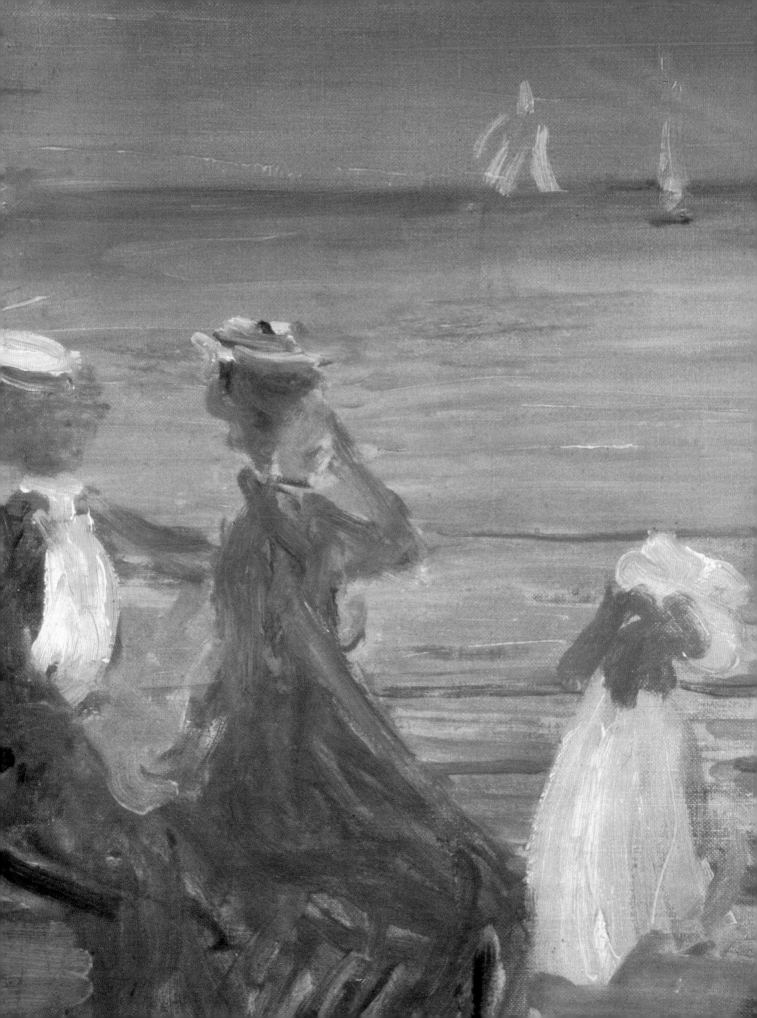

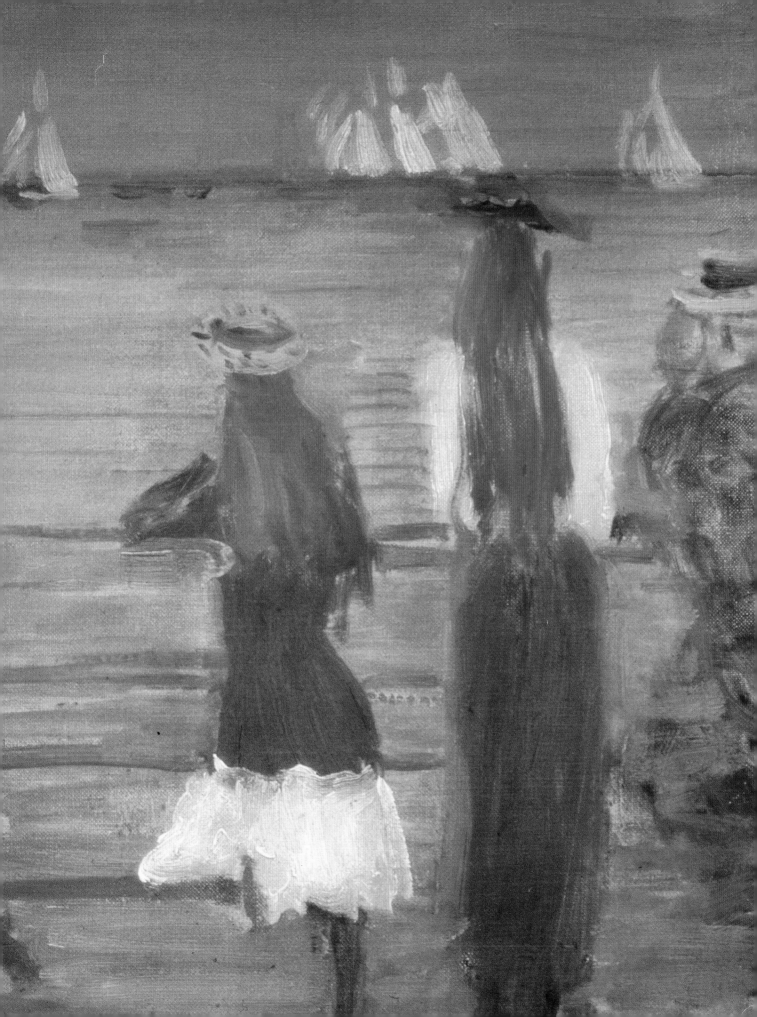

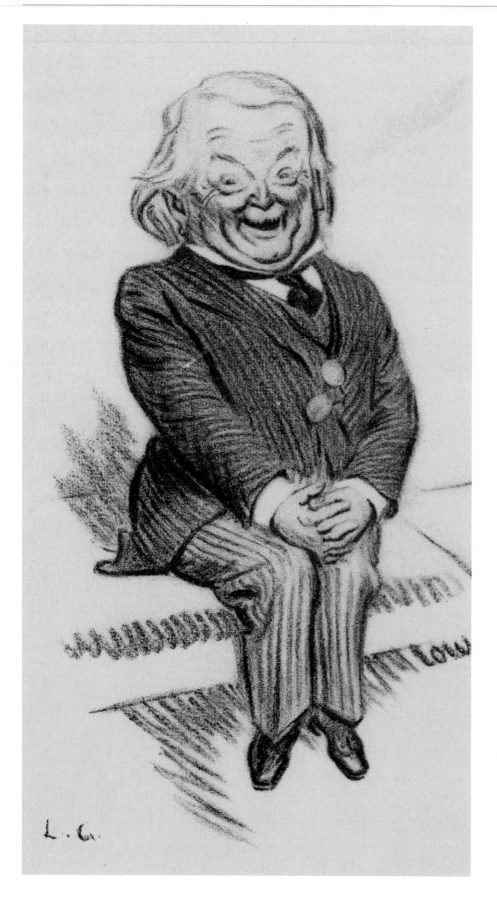

Fig. 93. Unusually long hair for a statesman — David Lloyd George, caricature by Low 1928

Fig. 94. (opposite) The mannish style as found in the demi-monde of Paris. Amedeo Modigliani, *The Amazon*, 1909 (private collection)

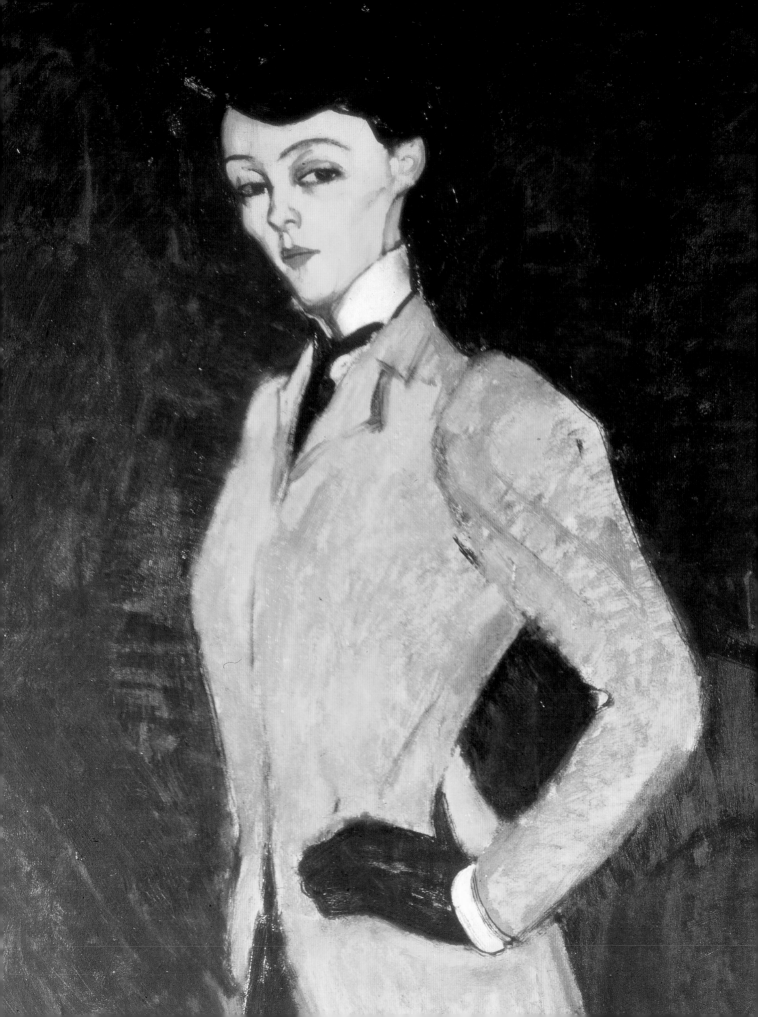

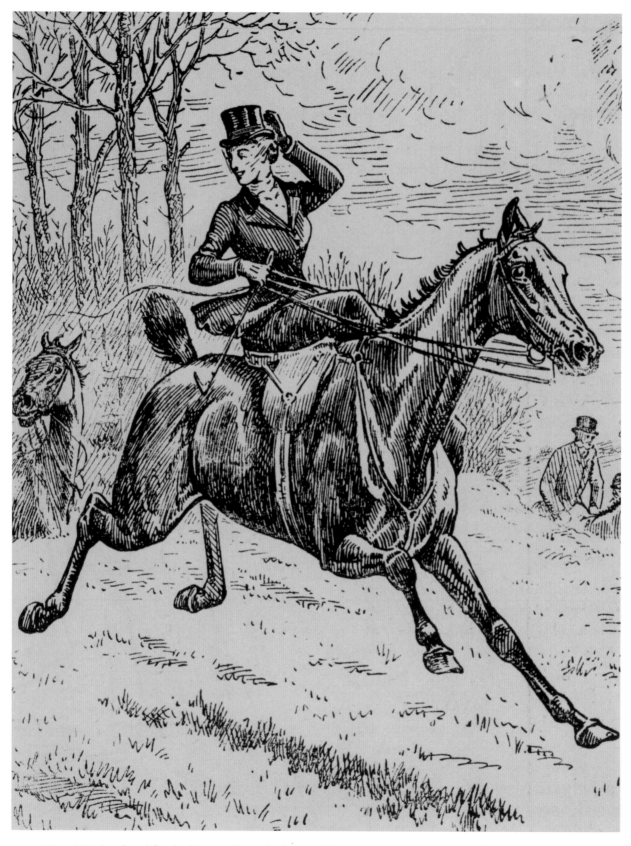

FIG. 95. One hand for the horse and one for hair and hat. From a cartoon, c. 1900 (author's collection)

However, the young girl in fg. 98 shows that long hair could be worn with charming abandon on a bicycle, but only if you were young enough. Most, however, would have to wait patiently for a new era.

The catalyst towards this impending change in female hairstyles was surely a new-found sense of independence. This applied not to just a few outstanding individuals but to the whole of womankind and is exemplified by the Suffragette movement, the marchers seeking votes for women. These were invariably well-dressed, well-hatted ladies, all with abundant hair - but this was surely a deliberate ploy to emphasise their respectability and conformity. Fashions would change when they had their way. The scissors would be out.

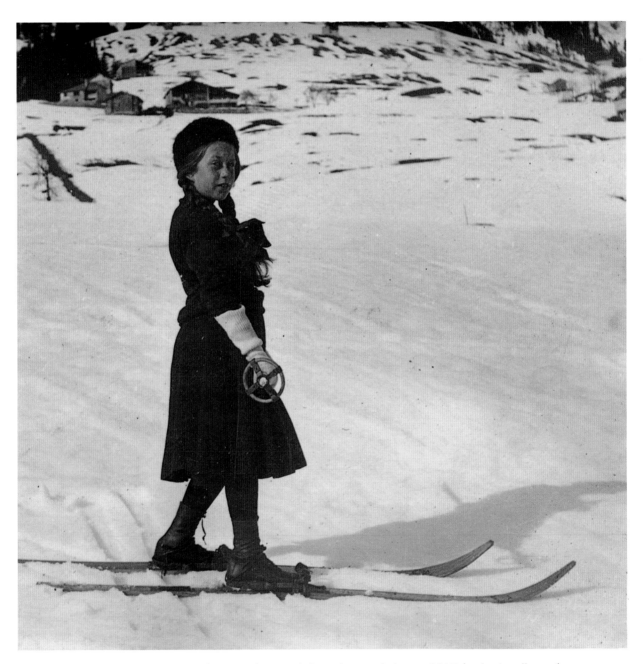

FIG. 96. Marjorie Grigsby goes skiing with hat, plaits and skirt, c. 1905 (author's collection)

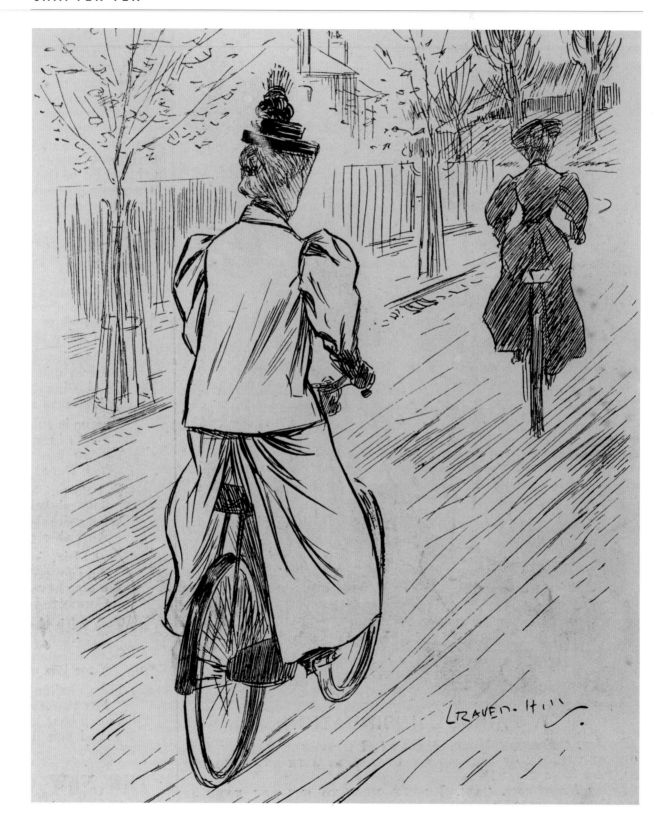

FIG. 97. Hats, veils, high-piled hair and flowing skirts hamper the budding cyclist.
From a cartoon, c. 1900 (author's collection)

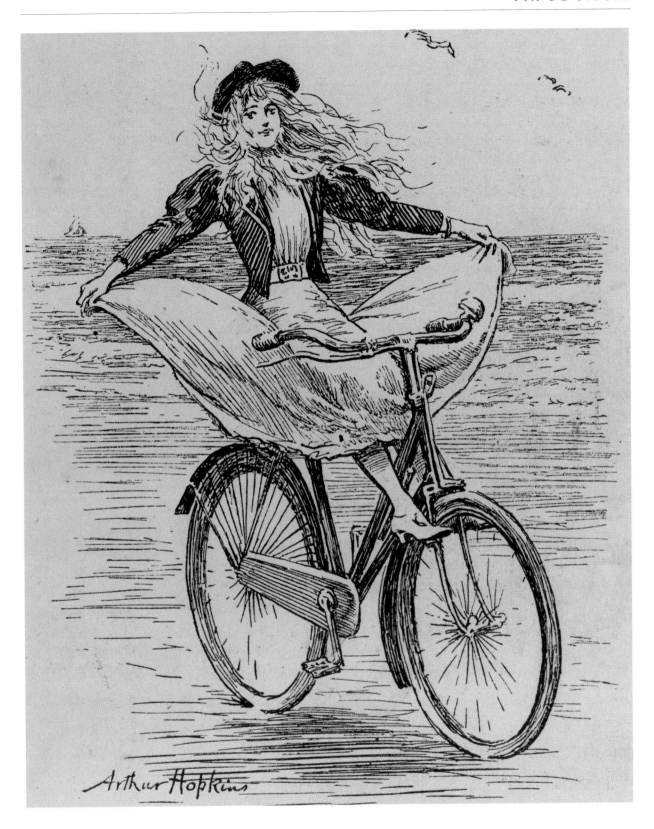

Fig. 98. Contrastingly casual — the freedom of the young.
From a cartoon, c. 1900 (author's collection)

WAR AND PEACE, THEN WAR AGAIN

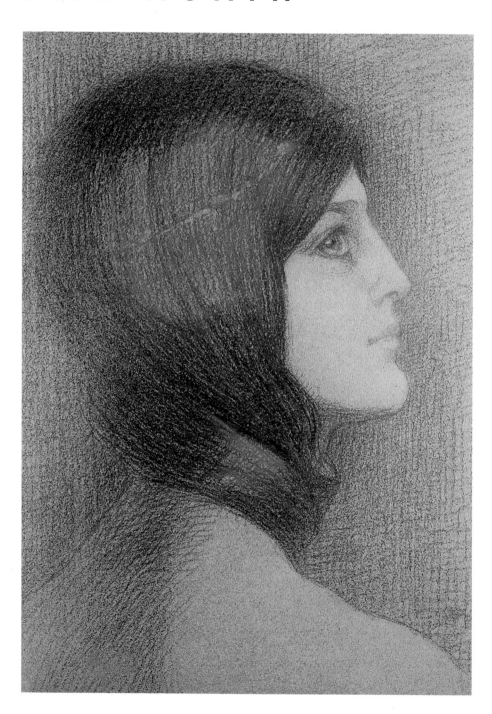

FIG. 99. The short look with long hair, inspired by a pilot's flying helmet. Armand Point, *Portrait of a Woman* (Whitford & Hughes, London)

I t was not just suffragettes who were on the march; soldiers were marching too, onward as to war – the First World War, to them the 'Great War'.

Surely distinctly war-inspired is the hairstyle seen in fig. 99. The girl's very long hair, wound around her neck and under her chin, gives the illusion of being short and close-fitting. It looks for all the world like the leather aviator's helmet of the time. As in the Napoleonic Wars, so a century later, as nations emerged from the Great War, hair was often worn not necessarily short but designed to give the impression of being so. So it is that the woman in fig. 100, though doubtless still able to let her hair down to her waist, has it plaited to either side and rolled up over both ears. From the imagery of the aviator, we have come to the imagery of the telephonist. It is almost as if she is wearing the two earpieces that were part of the stock-in-trade of the girls at the telephone exchange – new technology inspiring new fashions.

At this time it was not uncommon for a woman to keep her hair hidden, perhaps rolled at the back into a black scarf. Her front hair, loosely curled, and the hairs at the nape of her neck would be all that showed. Alternatively, she might have the front of her hair cut in a severe fringe, low over the eyebrows, with the hair to either side cut similarly severely over her ears. Yet her back hair might remain uncut, and be piled up like ice cream perching on a cone. Fashion was edging very

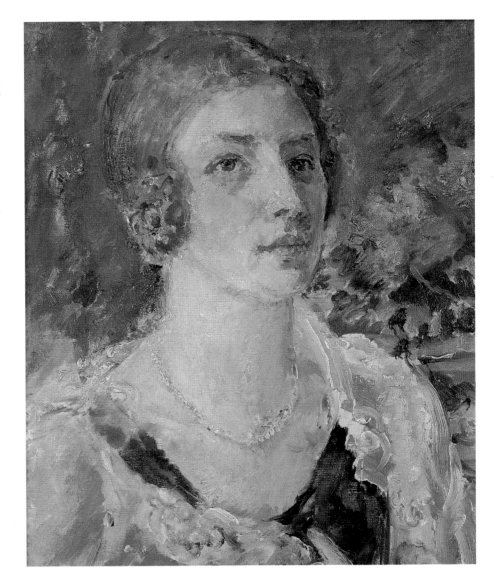

FIG. 100. The short look again – this time with coiled plaits over the ears, reminiscent of a telephonist's headphones. Ethel Walker, *The Lace Wrap* (Oldham Art Gallery, Lancashire)

cautiously towards the short haircut for women. In the 1800s women had been bolder than they were now in the early 1920s. Now there seemed to be no Madame Recamier to make the short style respectable. Quite how difficult it was proving for young women of this era to take the plunge – or, rather, seize the scissors – is illustrated by a story recently told by Kathleen Hale, author of the *Orlando* children's books, who recalled that she only narrowly missed being expelled from Reading University when she had her hair cut short.

Part of the stigma attached to short hair stemmed from its association with lesbianism. but also from the fact that peasant girls, particularly in Brittany and the Balkans, had their hair cut for sale, almost like an agricultural crop. In the entry under 'Hair' in the *Encyclopaedia Britannica* of 1911 it was recorded that: 'In the south of France the cultivation and sale of heads of hair by peasant girls is a common practice; and

The severity of the cut could be relieved with a side parting, which a few years before would have been condemned as outrageously masculine

hawkers attend fairs for the special purpose of engaging in this traffic.' The entry went on to say that 'scarcely any such "raw material" is obtained in the United Kingdom except in the form of ladies' combings'.

Kathleen Hale's crime, surely, was not so much that she cut her hair, but that she did so in order to sell it to defray her student expenses, hardly the action of a 'lady'. However, what Kathleen Hale had done for money, many women were now – almost literally – itching to do for pleasure. In Paris in 1922 models were taking the plunge by having their hair 'bobbed'. Shortly afterwards, Irene Castle made the style fashionable in the United States, and by 1925 Julia Hoyt had reported reading that every day, day after day, two thousand American women were having their locks shorn.

However, if 'Delilah' had had her way, as we have seen, it could all have happened sixty years before, at least on the Confederate side in the American Civil War. Presumably unaware of 'Delilah's' earlier call for women to sacrifice their hair in the Confederate cause, a certain New York barber, Signor Raspenti, claimed that he had

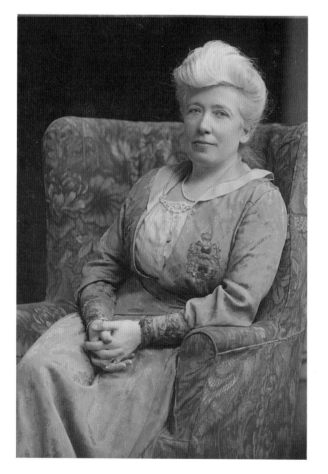

FIG. 101. An old fashioned mother – Gertrude Grigsby. photo c. 1918 (author's collection)

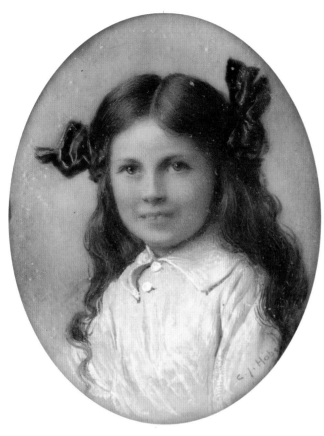

While the bob was essentially a classless style, in England it became very much the badge of high society

Fig. 102. — and her young daughter Joan as a girl. miniature on ivory, c. 1918 (author's collection)

started the craze for the 'bob' when a well-known female artist had demanded that he cut her hair short at least ten years previously. He now reckoned that there were not many more heads of hair available to be sacrificed, calculating that already ninety per cent of young women and fifty per cent of their elders had taken to the bob already. The daring style, slow in coming, had finally resulted in a whole avalanche of hair on to the barber's floor.

While the bob was essentially a classless style, in England it became very much the badge of high society. It was synonymous with the flapper, the giddy short-haired, tight-bosomed and short-skirted teenager dancing the night away. An unfortunate girl who had just had her hair similarly bobbed was told she must grow it

again when she applied for a job below stairs at Shugborough, Lord Lichfield's house. This was because one of the family had just had hers similarly cut. As the unfortunate would-be follower of fashion recalled in a recent BBC interview, she should have known better than to imitate her superiors.

This, too, was the age of the cigarette, something that no lady would have been seen smoking in public before the war. The habit somehow goes with short hair, since long hair can be easily singed and the smell of smoke can linger in its curls. Though it would have been frowned on before the war, few were scandalised now by the sight of a woman smoking. However, there were those who railed against the loss of long hair, citing in their aid St Paul's first letter to the Corinthians 11:6, where it says that it is 'a shame for a woman to be shorn or shaven'. To be bobbed or to have a 'garçon' or an Eton crop – or indeed the Titus style of the early nineteenth century – was, they argued, to be shorn and therefore to be shamed.

The severity of the cut could be relieved with a side parting, which a few years before would have been condemned as outrageously masculine. Having the hair shingled likewise restored something of the feminine to the short-haired female. The permanent wave had been introduced by Monsieur Marcelle in Paris as long ago as 1872. Now, with short hair in vogue, the attractiveness of introducing crisp waves and curls close to the scalp made full use of his and subsequent forms of 'perm'.

Thus it was that the society lady, having escaped the necessity of having a maid put up her hair, and the quandary, night after night, as to how best to dress it, had really only exchanged one tyranny for another. This was because she now had the new task of keeping her hair regularly cut and waved. These were changing times maybe, but no less lucrative for those whose business was the care of hair.

In the schoolroom, the society hostess made sure that her daughters still had long hair. Later she would permit them to have it cut, in just the same sort of rite of passage as had once been the moment when hair was first 'put up'. Both were a preliminary to that other

Despite the term 'Eton Crop' with its allusion to the well-known boys' school, these short haircuts were boyish but not like any a boy would usually have

strange society ritual, 'coming out'. The mother would look with some nostalgia at her daughter's flowing hair, enjoying the sight of it while revelling in the freedom of her own short cut. My own mother obtained that freedom while she was away at school, under the pretext of safety. She wrote home to break the news to her parents, explaining that her long hair had proved a hazard when it had nearly caught fire on a hot radiator – an implausible excuse in a world where, shortly, excuses would hardly be necessary. Her mother (fig. 101) must have grieved that the long haired little girl of the school room (fig. 102) has lost her crowning glory and joined the bobbed brigade (fig 103).

For the society hostess and the giddy flapper, style was everything. For the young woman away from home for the first time, the attraction perhaps was simply that of playing the tomboy. Despite the term 'Eton crop' with its allusion to the well-known boys' school, these short haircuts were boyish but not like any a boy would usually have.

Just as the bob had first taken hold in America, so more romantic antidotes to it were now, likewise, to flow eastwards across the Atlantic. The styles were imported both in films from Hollywood and on the heads of the film stars who appeared in them as they descended the gangways of the great Cunard liners at Southampton. The bob symbolised the independence that women had achieved, first by making themselves indispensable on the Home Front and behind the lines in the First World War and then by gaining the vote. Now came the introduction of new, less stark styles via the 'silver screen'. These, by contrast, came as a reaction to the Wall Street crash and the depression of the early 'thirties and would, in time, be such as to quicken the hearts of young pilot officers.

This softer glamour was perhaps personified by the film star Joan Crawford. Her swept-back hair had no parting and was 'permed' over her ears and at the back of her head. The style hinted at the equally flattering, but more cumbersome, longer styles of pre-bob times.

A drawing illustrating underwear (fig. 104) epitomises this more flowing look. Some women now again wore rather more hair at the back, often in the form of a 'transformation' – as hairpieces were somewhat euphemistically described. While the 1911 *Encyclopaedia Britannica*, as we have seen, recorded a great commerce in hair, particularly from the south of France, the 1948 edition made no such reference. From where, then, did these 'transformations' come? The answer is probably from the wearer's own head. Having first had her 'bob', and then grown her hair into some variety of long-short style, she could always add to it at party time with something made from the hair she had originally shed on the hairdresser's floor, perhaps some years before. If anyone dared to ask, she could truthfully say that, yes, all the hair on her head was hers, as Lady Hamilton

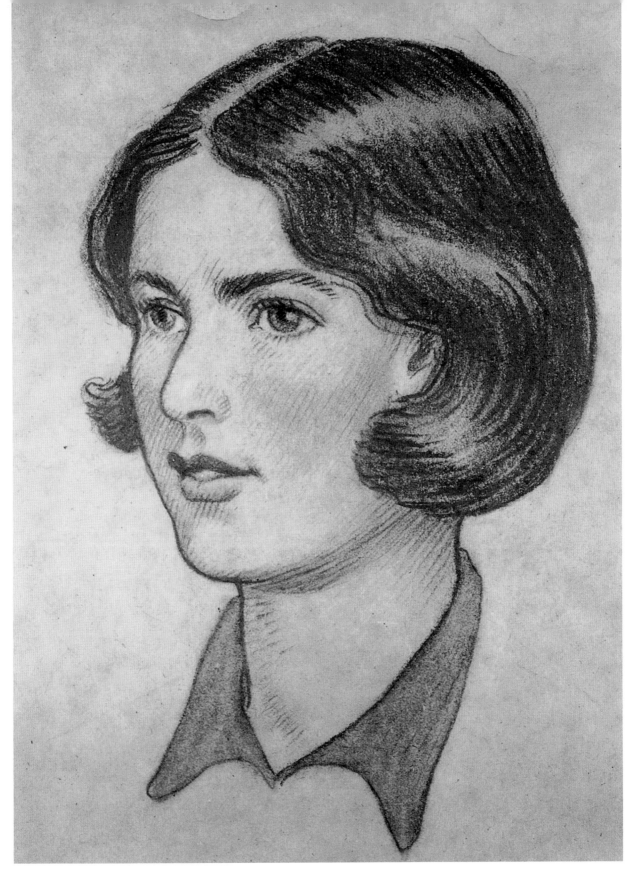

Fig. 103. — and as a young woman with her hair bobbed in a less graceful post-war world.
Joan Grigsby, 1934, drawing by Stanley Rogers (author's collection).

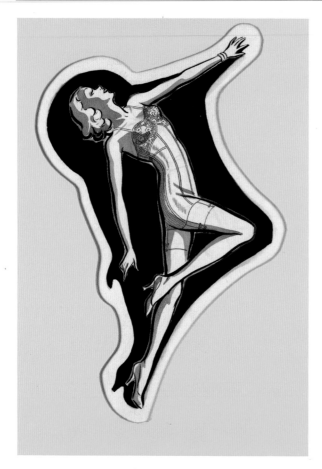

FIG. 104. An English example of the softer, longer Hollywood look. Drawing for an underwear advertisement c.1935 (author's collection)

Brylcreemed pilots whose return could not be guaranteed. Troops had to be entertained, too, with a glimpse of glamour and some stars were universal enough to transcend wartime barriers, such as the universally admired German idol, Marlene Dietrich.

Defiant of the incendiary bombs landing on her roof, my grandmother would sit in her south coast drawing room turning not a hair of her elaborate Edwardian coiffure, worn no differently in 1940 from the way she had worn it in 1904. How different from my mother! As an Air Force wife she was an age away both from herself as a long-haired little girl in her nursery and how she would look had she followed in her mother's time honoured example. Having a side parting with the hair left to grow longer over the ears, so that it could be curled over them, was her own distinctive evolution of the bob that she first acquired in the 1920s

Defiant of the incendiary bombs landing on her roof, my grandmother would sit in her south coast drawing room turning not a hair of her elaborate Edwardian coiffure, worn no differently in 1940 from the way she had worn it in 1904

might have done over a century before.

The mention of quickening the heart of a young pilot officer heralds the sad fact that, in the brief space of twenty years between the arrival of the bob and the firm establishment of Hollywood as a leader of fashion, the world had again entered into war. The picture in fig. 105 is said to date from 1939. If so, it was surely anticipating the wartime years. Certainly, the woman's lit-up face starkly framed by the roll of dark hair on her forehead and the curve of dark hair to either side of her temples, set against a dark sky in an open landscape, leads one to imagine that she is searching the skies for a returning aircraft. When life was short and precious, sweethearts on the ground had every reason to make themselves as attractive as possible for the young

(heralded by that ominous letter she wrote from school). Here she is seen in mid-war, the model of a dutiful air force wife (fig. 106) and, for good measure, here is the companion portrait of my father. (fig. 107) demonstrating the severe cut essential for all men (but not as severe as the crew cut favoured by his American colleagues). My mother's side curls were kept in place

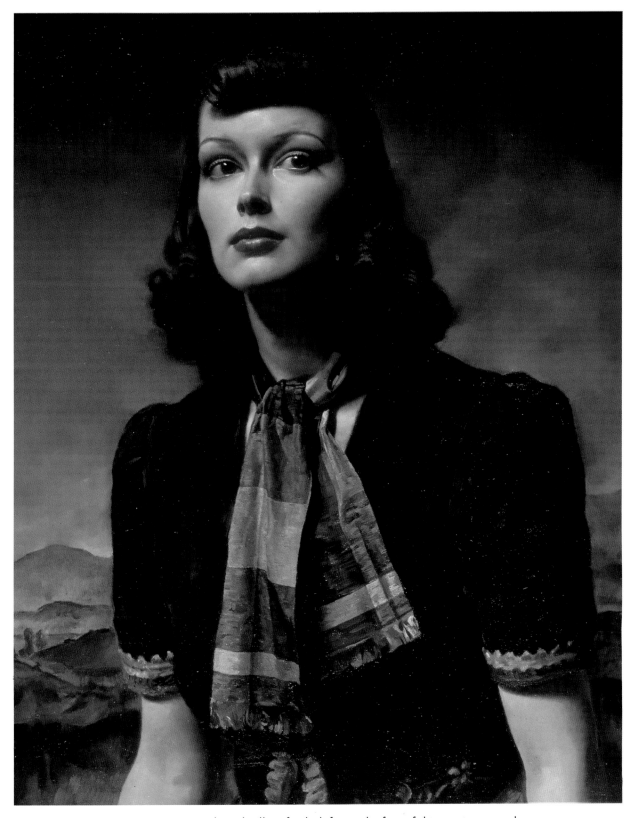

FIG.105. Lustrous curls and rolling forelock frame the face of this wartime sweetheart.
Gerald Leslie Brockhurst, *By the Hills*, c.1939 (Hull City Museums and Art Galleries, Ferens Art Gallery)

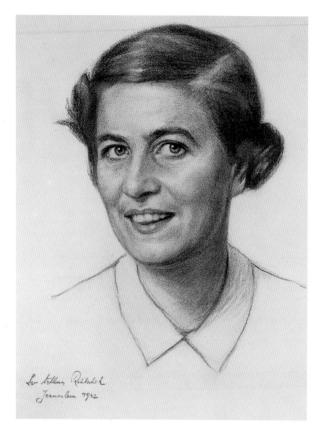

FIG. 106. Wartime airforce wife with her variation of the bob. *Joan Bryer (née Grigsby)*, drawing by Leo Arthur Robitschek, Jerusalem 1942 (author's collection).

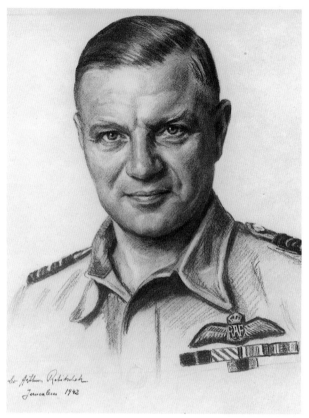

FIG. 107. – and her husband with appropriately severe haircut essential in the armed services (and civvy street too). *Peter Bryer*, drawing by Leo Arthur Robitscheck, Jerusalem 1942 (author's collection)

over the ears by a kirby grip apiece. She offered my brother and me a penny for every one we could find. We soon saw the good sense of buying them by the packet to sell to her individually every time she ran out. She was to continue to wear her hair in this fashion well into the 1950s. Not for her the long-short look of 1930s Hollywood, or the Paris of 1949 (fig. 108) as France once more emerged from the austerities of war.

FIG. 108. The short-long look on a post-war Parisienne.
Moise Kisling, *Portrait of Madame Martin*
(private collection)

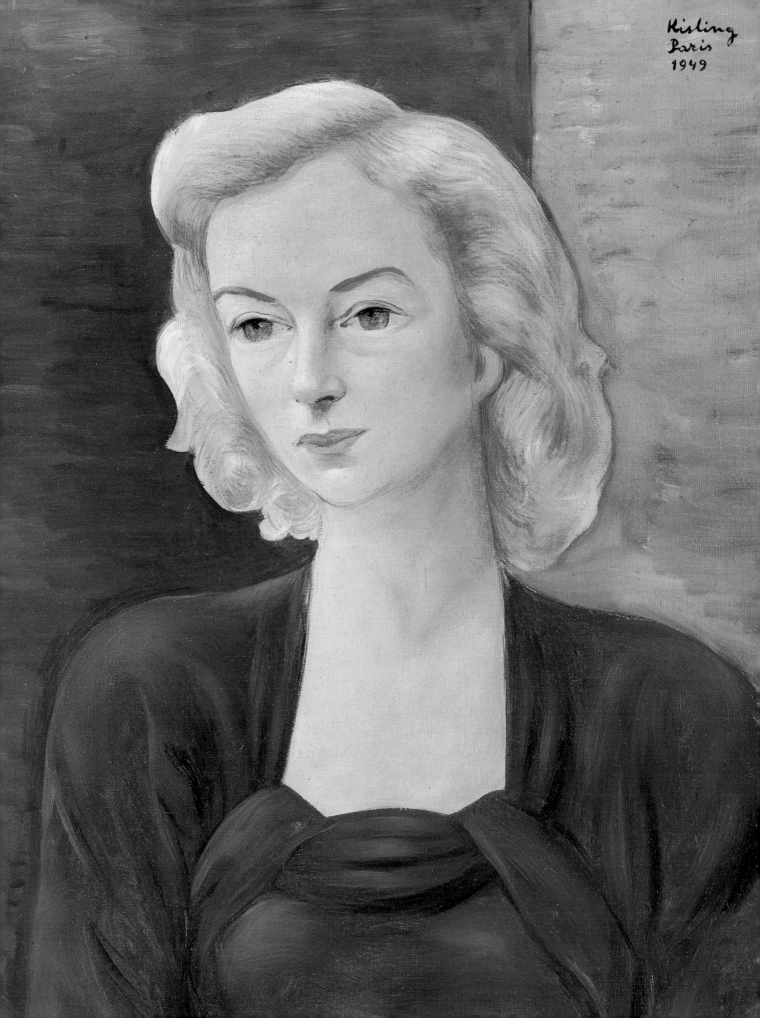

BRAVE NEW WORLD

FIG. 109. The first short-haired princess? Harry Watson, *HM The Queen as Princess Elizabeth* (private collection/Ackermann and Johnson Ltd, London)

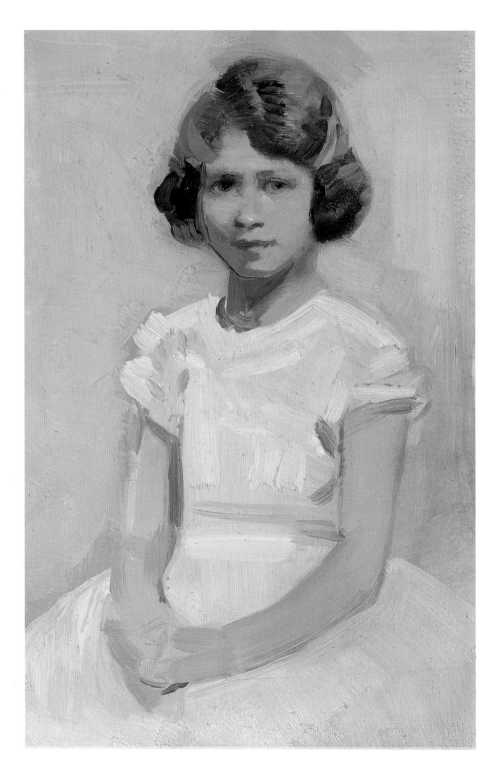

A mother with her short, bobbed hair might well keep her daughter in pigtails. Such a fashion in children could date from before the Second World War or after (or indeed during) and could equally well come from Austria, the land of *Heidi*, or America, the home of Judy Garland and *The Wizard of Oz*, as from the England of *Swallows and Amazons*. But Amazon Nancy, remember, had just the one pigtail, pirate fashion – a tomboy's way to wear long hair, which persists to this day.

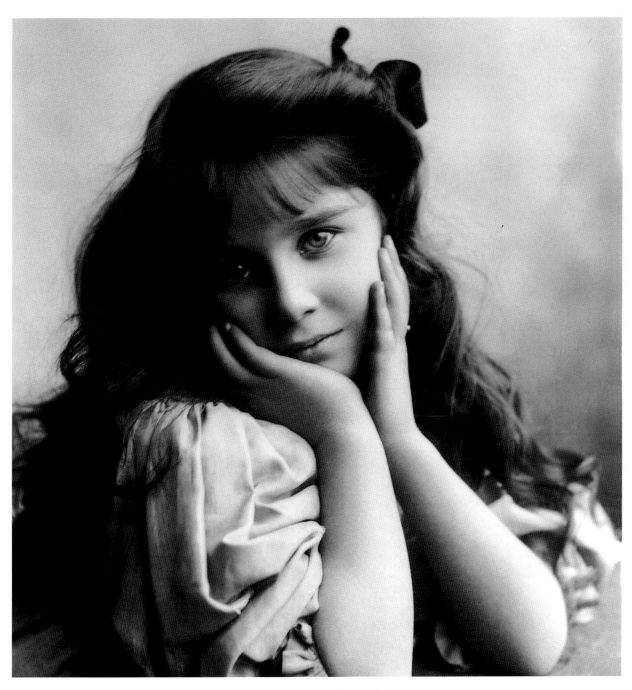

FIG. 110. The Queen's mother at the same age.
Lady Elizabeth Bowes-Lyon (now HM Queen Elizabeth, The Queen Mother)

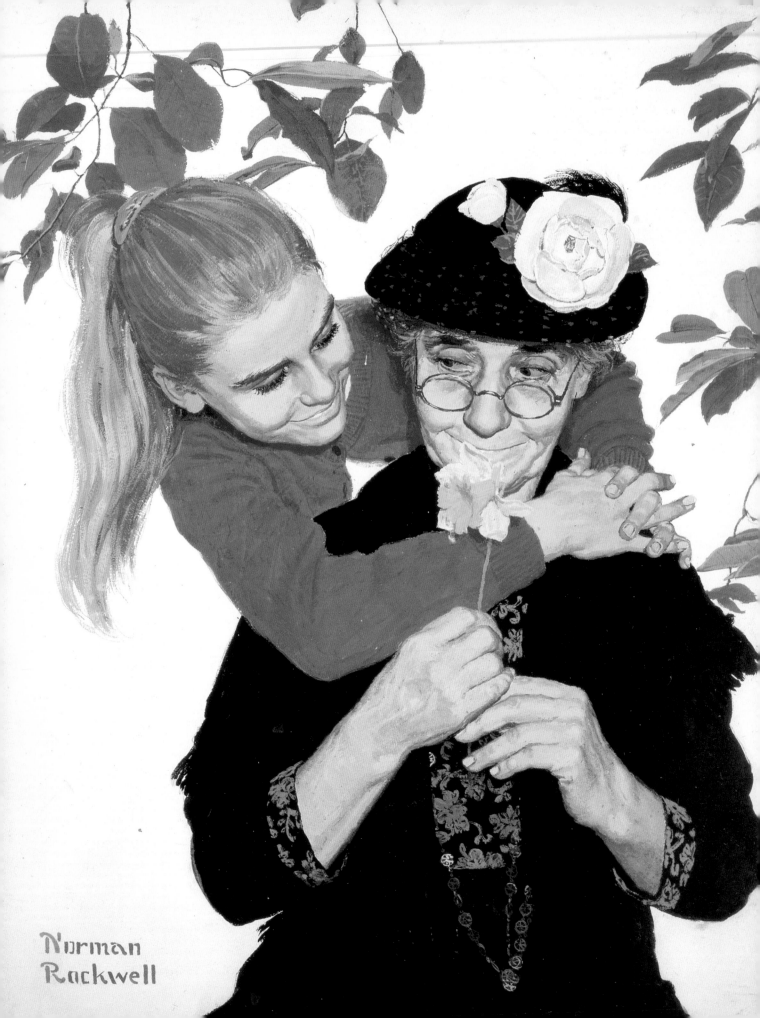

However, by contrast, the girl in fig. 109 has short hair. Known to us all, this is Princess Elizabeth, now Queen Elizabeth II. She must surely have been the first short-haired princess since the days before Cleopatra. Her parents were somewhat avant garde to give her such a relatively short hairstyle as a child, particularly when you compare her picture with that of her mother at the same age (fig. 110). It was a style, however, that was surely well chosen. Not aggressively short and very definitely feminine, it has proved, with remarkably little change, to be as appropriate for Her Majesty today as it was when she was a little girl. Not for her the great change in hairstyle between youth and maturity of those two other great monarchs, Victoria and her own namesake, the first Elizabeth.

If there is a prevailing hairstyle in her own Elizabethan age, it comes not from her example but from popular culture, and from the west side of the Atlantic rather than the east: it is, surely, the ponytail. Adopted by all ages and worn in varying lengths, this simplest of styles is worn high at the back of the head. At its most basic, this style panders to the little girl's desire to empathise with her pony. It also evokes the world of bobby socks and A-line skirts. The pony tail was an essential part of a girl's equipment, to toss about while dancing in the rock-and-roll years of the 1950s. A good American example of the ponytail comes from that master of paintings observing American culture, Norman Rockwell (fig. 111). Here the hair is all of one length pulled smoothly back. However the ponytail can also go with a fringe and a parting across the head behind it. The ponytail is nothing if not universal, from Russia to the United States and from New Zealand to Japan.

But why should it be so much a symbol of our time, rather than timeless? Perhaps it is because the second generation of women, following the bobbing revolution, had either never learnt how to plait hair or did not care

FIG. 111. The ponytail, symbol of a post-war world. Norman Rockwell, *A Young Girl and her Grandmother* (Bonhams, London)

to do so, finding it quicker and easier to tie back their daughters' hair in a ponytail instead. A more likely reason, however, is the advent of the humble rubber band. Prior to its arrival, a plait had to be tied with a silk bow or sewn in place with needle and cotton. The ponytail cannot easily be sewn into place, since, unlike a plait, the cotton has nothing with which to intertwine. The alternative of a silk bow would come adrift very easily and, in any case, does not look streetwise to modern eyes. An elastic band looks simple, holds securely, and is easy to either slip on direct or twist into a figure of eight. So the queue of the eighteenth century becomes the ponytail of today, minus the hassle of

The pony tail was an essential part of a girl's equipment, to toss about while dancing in the rock-and-roll years of the 1950s

requiring a parent or servant to secure it. It has become somewhat androgynous, too, since the 1960s – reasonably enough, since it was a male style in the first place. Now, in the twenty-first century, male advertising executives and city dealers wear their ponytails over their dark suits without raising a doorman's eyebrow.

However, if the swing of the ponytail was to go from the female to the male, there was also to be a two-way traffic in hairstyles between men and women. The girl in her bobby socks and A-line skirt, rock'n'rolling away, did not have her fantasy sufficiently fulfilled by dreaming that she was dancing with the king himself, Elvis Presley. She actually wanted to look like him. With his hair longer at the front, worn in a quiff and with a kiss curl or two hanging over the forehead, Elvis (dare it be said?) had taken a step from the male towards the female, though his extravagant sideburns (and much more besides) confirmed his masculinity. The excuse for such departures from the strict very short back and sides of the post-war years had its roots in the Teddy boy movement, seeking to recreate the dandy of the Edwardian period. The surprise was that women should follow suit, in homage to their idol.

While some girls might have been sacrificing their ponytails at the end of the 'fifties in order to emulate a pop-star idol, others most definitely did not. In 1982, in retrospect, Ann Barr and Peter York identified an enduring style beloved of middle- and upper-class traditionalists on both side of the Atlantic. Its Mecca was not Elvis Presley's Gracelands but the streets around London's Sloane Square. These were the Sloane Rangers and, in the 'fifties and 'sixties, the female of the species

> **If there was one characteristic which defined the female Sloane hairstyle, it was that it obeyed the typical mother's practical exhortation to 'keep it out of your eyes, dear'**

was seldom without her so-called Alice band, which must surely also be a symbol of the twentieth century. It is named after Lewis Carroll's Alice, not so much the little girl upon whom Carroll based his stories but as she appears in Tenniel's illustrations. While it is true that a small Victorian girl might well have had a ribbon passed over the top of her head and behind the ears, to be tied beneath her hair at the nape, this would not be very secure. It is no surprise that the real Alice is seen in photographs with a fringe and no ribbon. The Alice band of today, by contrast, is horseshoe-shaped. It does not circle under the hair, even if it appears to do so. Simply spanning from ear to ear, it takes advantage of modern plastic materials that can be made to fit the head closely, so as to be secure but not uncomfortable. The modern woman, therefore, can have shoulder-length or longer hair, but be able to keep it controlled with a minimum of fuss by holding it back, away from

her face, with an Alice band. No true Sloane, up until the seventies, would have been without at least two of these hair bands, one covered in navy blue and the other in black velvet.

If there was one characteristic which defined the female Sloane hairstyle, it was that it obeyed the typical mother's practical exhortation to 'keep it out of your eyes, dear'. An aid to this was and is the other universal female Sloane accessory, the headscarf. The inspiration here does not come from a story about a small Victorian girl but the wartime economy of dispensing with a hat in favour of a scarf, be you a cleaner scrubbing the front doorstep or a princess riding in Windsor Great Park. However, if you think that this simple utilitarian fashion would tend to make everyone equal, you are mistaken. For the true Sloane Ranger, the scarf must be designed by Hermès and tied beneath the chin like a guardsman's chinstrap.

Christine Keeler in fig. 112 is not wearing an Alice band, a scarf, or (it would seem) anything else, apart from the back of a chair. But her shoulder-length hair could be easily controlled by one or the other, if circumstances demanded it. It is worn freely in a way not seen in previous centuries. The reason why such hairstyles are now relatively universal is the increased availability of shampoo and blow dryers. The *Encyclopaedia Britannica* of 1946 recommended that one should wash one's hair once a fortnight. The twenty-first-century woman washes it almost daily. Hair such as Christine Keeler's could be easily washed and blow-dried so that, given an hour's notice, it need never look straggly, greasy or lank. No one need accuse her of having dirty hair, as they did her early nineteenth-century counterpart, Emma Hamilton.

The simple cut and 'wash and go' (to quote a shampoo catchphrase) was not for everyone, however. Contemporary with Christine Keeler's heyday, the early

FIG. 112. Medium-length hair can be worn freely in an age of shampoos and blow dryers.
Lewis Morley, bromide print of Christine Keeler, 1963

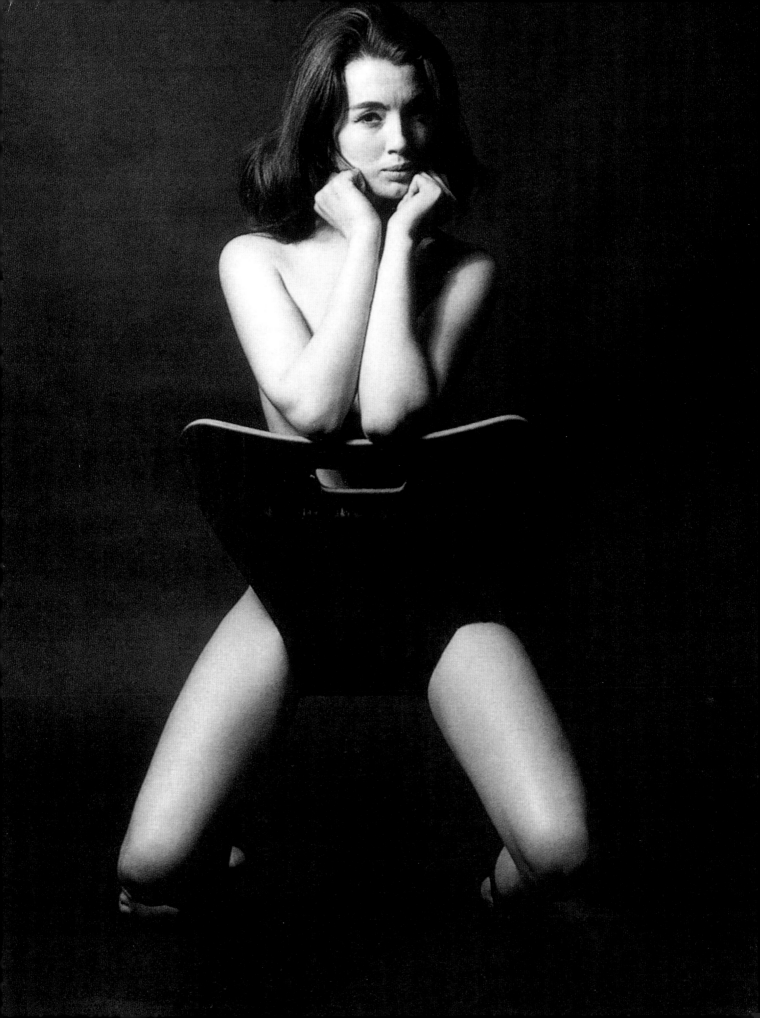

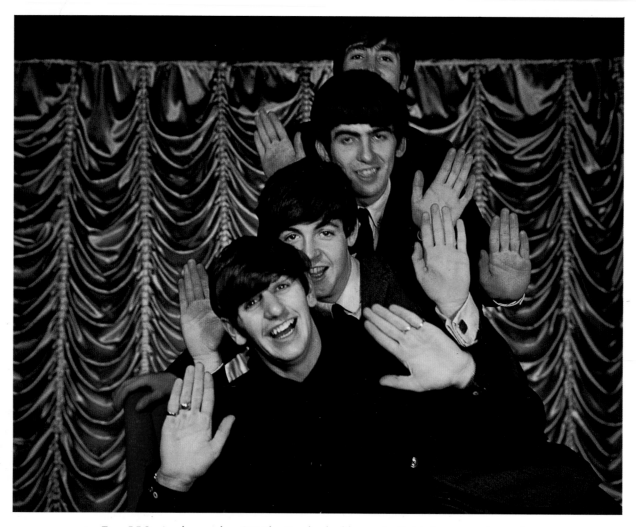

FIG. 113. Lowbrow rules, OK! The Beatles had an unrivalled influence on hairstyles in the second half of the twentieth century (photo Aquarius)

1960s, was that remarkable confection, the beehive hairdo. Unlike the extraordinary, towering concoctions of the middle of the fifteenth century in Italy and the eighteenth century in France and England, the beehives of the late 'sixties and early 'seventies were not usually subject to verminous infestation. Light pads could be used to support them, but more importantly they benefited from another new invention – lacquer in aerosol cans. A girl could walk with confidence with hair piled as high as a guardsman's busby, once sprayed solid with an appropriate lacquer. Going to bed, however, was another matter. One had to be careful to lie on one's side, as Sandie Shaw recalled recently, shortly before her death. A headscarf over a beehive, though necessary

on a windy night when dashing from a taxi to the theatre door, was hardly a thing of beauty, looking for all the world like a tarpaulin over an old-fashioned haystack.

Aesthetics apart, the practicality of running to a theatre on a windy night, to say nothing of obstructing the view of those behind you once seated safely inside, could lead to your abandoning the beehive style. In preference, again crossing the genders, a girl might be influenced by what she saw on the stage in front of her, particularly if it was the 1963 production of the musical *Oliver*. In the 1960s girls might well have been seeking to capture the waif-like looks of young Oliver Twist's ragged, short, urchin cut.

Meanwhile, in the cinema, the more female but

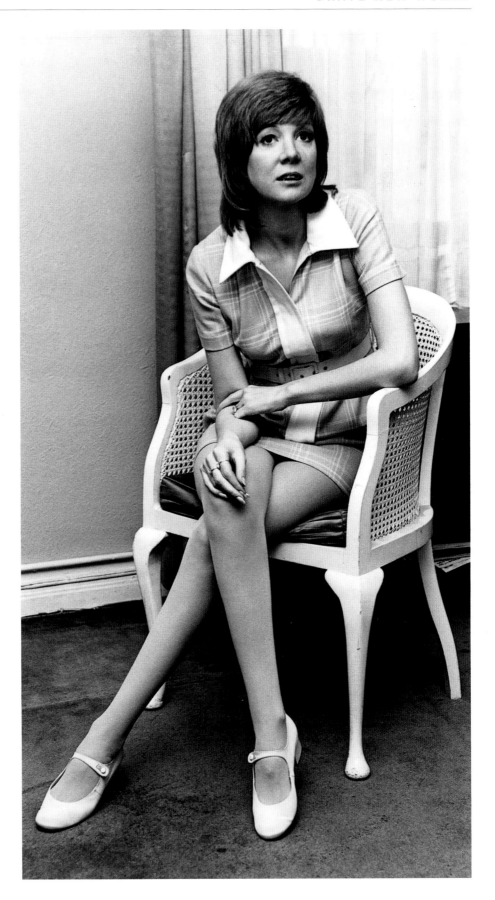

Fig. 114. Cilla Black in February 1970 — Liverpool's one-girl answer to its most famous male quartet, The Beatles (and just as enduring), complete with her own version of the Beatle haircut. (photo Universal Pictorial Press)

equally short cut of Julie Andrews as she appeared in *The Sound of Music* was to be a similarly strong influence. It was short because the character of the nun that she played had been shorn as part of the nun's rejection of the sexually glamorous. With her head in a wimple, the length of her hair would have been unknown. However, dancing bare-headed over the Alps with her young charges, that sexual glamour was, if anything, emphasised. The long-haired girl gazing up at her nun-turned-nanny would obviously wish to emulate her role model and have her hair cut likewise. That did not come into the story of the film, but it certainly had an effect on women watching it.

However, nun-like or boy-like, it hardly mattered. The Beatles' mophead haircuts (fig. 113) remind one not of nuns but of pageboys, or, rather more maturely,

Prince Machiavelli (see fig. 27). In 1964 they took New York by storm. It was not so much the length of the hair – long for a man and short for a woman by standards current at the time – but the fact that there was no parting and it hung so low over the eyes as to obliterate the brow. Elizabeth I plucked her forehead to enhance a look of great intelligence, making her (literally) 'highbrow'. The Beatles, by contrast, centuries on were literally 'lowbrow', their looks belying their intelligence and their enduring art. Their importance, in hair fashion terms, cannot be overemphasised. What probably started as a public relations gimmick to get noticed turned, instead, into a long delayed flow of fashion from east to west across the Atlantic (rather than vice versa) and, in social terms, from working-class Liverpool to the highest ranks of society. This latter was the most

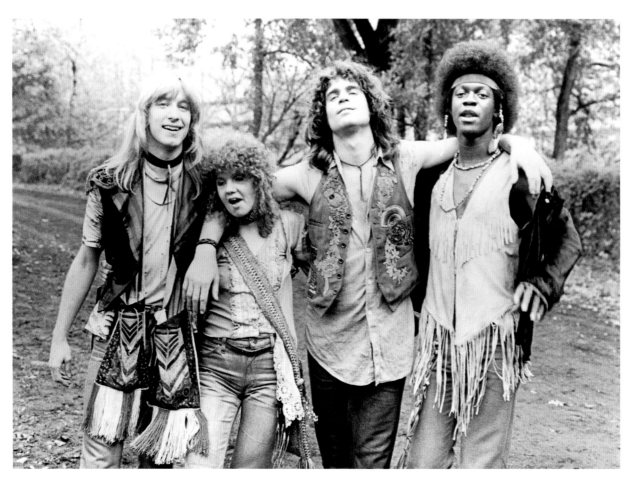

FIG. 115. Out in the open – from straight blond through to extravagantly frizzy Afro, four members of the cast of *Hair* span the full sexual and ethnic spectrum. (photo Aquarius)

remarkable. This was surely the first instance ever of a fashion spreading upwards through the classes rather than downwards. The Beatles' haircut was not to be an enduring style for men, not even for themselves. However, it was to be for women, particularly for that 'honorary' Beatle, their Liverpool contemporary Cilla Black (fig. 114). Her hair is longer at the back and sides but very similarly 'lowbrow' at the front. If a low brow indicates lack of intelligence, that is hardly borne out by her becoming, as she has, one of the highest-paid women of all time. But then, Prince Machiavelli and the Beatles were pretty bright too.

In terms of hairstyle, the Beatles were mild in comparison to the Rolling Stones with their long hair to the side and back, for which Mick Jagger actually sported a little frock to match when in concert in Hyde Park in 1969. Boys were now wearing their hair long so as not to be mistaken for their short-haired girlfriends. Girls, if they could afford it, would be going to Vidal Sassoon on both sides of the Atlantic, seeking an asymmetrical geometric cut or a version of the Beatle cut, carefully sculpted to skim the ears, the nape and the eyebrows. Such hairstyles were to complement the clothing styles of Mary Quant, she of the mini-skirt who famously (we are told) had her pubic hairs cut in the shape of a heart, bringing a new dimension to the word 'hairdressing'. It was her mini-skirt which, ironically, led to further mixing of the genders. It could not have flourished had self-supporting tights not taken over from stockings and suspender belts. As skirts shrank to little more than wide belts, one questioned: why wear a skirt at all? The unisex revolution was upon us and the first of the now universal unisex hairdressers began to emerge, one of the first being Sissors in Chelsea.

The importance of hair in this revolution was never made clearer than with the arrival in London from New York in 1968 of the musical aptly entitled *Hair*, in which one of the lyrics included the lines 'Hair like Jesus wore it / Hallelujah, I adore it'.

While nudity was the factor that tempted the audience into London's West End to see the show, it was the hair of the title, in all its variety, rather than bare flesh, which played the most important part. This

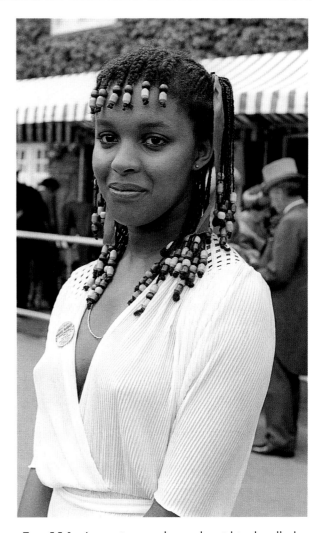

FIG. 116. A man in a top hat and a girl in dreadlocks — Enola Griffith, aged 19, proudly brings her own ethnic style to Royal Ascot in 1980. (photo Graham Morris, Hulton Getty)

was not regimented hair as in the case of the lookalike Beatles, but the hair of individual self-expression stemming from a flower-people's 'Be-in' in New York's Central Park. Fig. 115 shows four of the cast walking down an English country lane, fully clothed rather than naked in front of the footlights. From left to right, we have first blond hair, which a decade before would have been cut severely short on a man (embarrassed enough at being blond) but is here allowed its full luxuriance with ample length. Then comes curly hair, which even

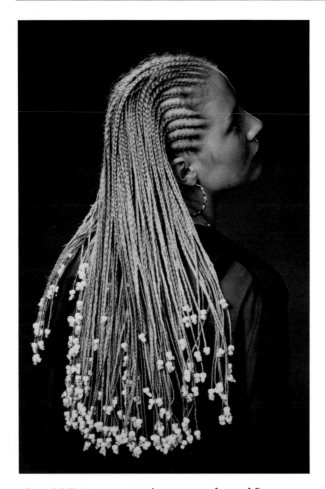

FIG. 117. Imitation is the sincerest from of flattery – you can have long, blonde hair in dreadlocks too. *Katie at Carl Hillwood.* (photo Richard Lines, Ringwood)

in dreadlocks, beaded at the ends. In her own way she is every bit as self-expressive as the gentleman in the morning coat and top hat behind her is in his.

Imitation is the sincerest form of flattery. We see it in fig. 115 where the fair-skinned girl is letting her curls grow in imitation of the Afro style of her dark-skinned companion. We see it again in fig. 119, where long and straight blonde hair, the nature of which does not require the discipline of tight plaiting, is nonetheless worn in dreadlocks in imitation of the girl's dark-skinned and

> Quantities of hair gel can be applied to make the hair stand up in spikes and a greater impact can be achieved with the addition of colour – green, orange, red, white or blue, according to choice

dark-haired contemporaries.

The Beatles and the Rolling Stones, though initially aiming to shock, were really 'mothers' boys' at heart, ready to be absorbed into the establishment, complete with their MBEs. The Sex Pistols, however, ten years on in 1976, really did set out to shock – in terms of language, sound and above all appearance. But even the punk movement, of which they were the archpriests, quickly became a tame part of the tourist scene, quite as likely to feature on London souvenirs as pictures of guardsmen or beefeaters. Undoubtedly, there could have been punk without the Sex Pistols. The style simply grew out of fashion's continuing need to test the boundaries.

The Mohican is the quintessential punk hairstyle, as inconvenient on the pillow as the beehive. As with dreadlocks, its antecedents are ethnic – this time not from the Afro community but from that of the American Indian. Its creation and maintenance are equally time-consuming, but it's all part of the tribal grooming ritual,

(as here) on a girl would previously have been suppressed and straightened, not least because of its Afro connotations, whereas here it is allowed to run riot. Next, a male brunette allows his hair something of the luxuriance not seen on a man since the days of celebrity highwaymen. And last but certainly not least, Afro hair that would once have been close-cropped or laboriously straightened is allowed to spread like a mushroom cloud ever outwards and upwards. From now on people would increasingly be allowed to make the most of hair's attributes and character, regardless of sex or race.

A charming example of this flowering of ethnic expression is shown in fig. 117. Here the nineteen-year-old Enola Griffith is attending Royal Ascot with her hair be the 'tribesman' English, American or African. Fashion, after all, never was supposed to be labour-saving. Children had long been intrigued by the hairstyle they had seen in Wild West movies and now, with the sanction which the punk movement gave them, they steeled themselves in adolescence to re-create the Mohican on their own heads. With delighted fascination they would watch as each side of the head was shaved, leaving a comb of floppy hair in the centre. And today's technology allows for further refinement not available to the native American. Quantities of hair gel can be applied to make the hair stand up in spikes and a greater impact can be achieved with the addition of colour – green, orange, red, white or blue, according to choice. However, even if the object was to shock your parents, the end result could be charming, as in fig. 118. Here

Adee has added purpose to the shaved sides of her head by having it adorned with an Aztec tattoo, which complements her brilliant red Mohican cockscomb. One day she may be a grandmother with her skull demurely covered in close white curls, but for the time being this child of the 1970s delights, rather than defies, the world with her exotic plumage.

In the late twentieth century an enduring style moved us one step on from the Mohican: that of the skinhead, again for both men and women. It surely dates back to Yul Brynner, whose head was famously shaved for the film *The King and I*. More recently the Irish singer Sinead O'Connor transformed her image overnight when the knee-length hair that she used to wear free, not up, was replaced not by a bob but by a totally shaved head. She had it shaved, she said, as a

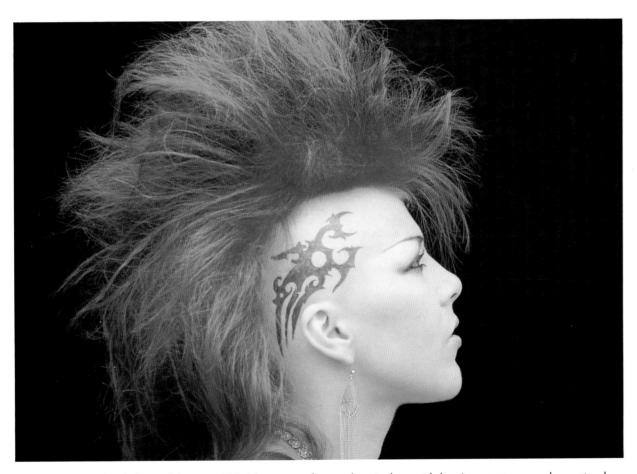

Fig. 118. Startlingly beautiful – in 1985 Adee personifies punk at its best with her Aztec tattoo complementing her Mohican haircut. (Tattoo by Lal Hardy, hair by Adee, photo Chris Wroblewski Skin Shows).

men drool over. Yet she must surely also have done it knowing of the frisson that extremes can bring and (if a woman is beautiful) the beauty there is in baldness. If, as a woman, she thought that she was doing something new, however, she was mistaken. One only has to look back to fig. 7 to remind oneself of this. That said, in the more recent past, the shaven-headed female has been seen as a figure of shame – in France the heads of collaborators were shaved after the World War II. Now female baldness is not unfamiliar. Indeed, in some it is temporarily inevitable as the result of chemotherapy. In others, shaving the head perhaps demonstrates sympathy and identity with those who have no choice,

> **By the end of the twentieth century wigs were again being worn more from necessity than in the interests of fashion, but often equally openly**

just as Marie Antoinette's courtiers shed some of their hair when she, after childbirth, lost much of hers. Who knows?

However, the shaved head is as time-consuming to maintain as a full head of hair, so that a girl may try it once but let it grow into what has now become an androgynous crew cut. Thus a blonde's head may look more like a field of stubble than one ripe for harvest.

Talk of shaved heads and crew cuts brings us back to a fashion for wigs. The wig saw a great revival in the 1960s, particularly with synthetic 'fun' wigs, sometimes in colours that anticipated the punks by a whole decade. The whole point was, however, that one could instantly be transformed and any shock induced could be as transient as you chose. The Beatles' arrival in New York gave rise to a massive market in Beatle wigs, to be worn once and then deposited on top of the wardrobe – to be mistaken perhaps, from time to time, for the family cat. Today it might be considered politically incorrect

that the more expensive human hair wigs should require that Italian and Balkan peasant girls be shorn in order to adorn the heads of the supposedly more sophisticated on either side of the Atlantic. The more realistic, however, would simply regard the sale of hair as being a good way in which a farmer's daughter could contribute a useful 'catch crop' to the family's economy. History repeating itself. In India such a sacrifice was made in any case for religious reasons, though rather than the priests burning the hair, the government set up a hair processing factory in Madras, which, by the end of the 1960s, was reported to be turning out some 12,000 wigs per month.

In the 1950s American girls were supplementing their own hair with falls of hair attached to a band. In the 1960s, with a fashion for more sculptural styles (fig. 119), the total wig had obvious advantages. So teased and lacquered was the whole ensemble that it was indeed more sculpted than cut or dressed. It could equally be one's own hair, the product of many hours in the hairdresser's chair, or a wig, capable of being tidied up in the hair salon while one went shopping. Whichever was the case, there was no longer any need for deception. By the end of the twentieth century wigs were again being worn more from necessity than in the interests of fashion, but often equally openly. Famously, Mo Mowlam, having lost her hair through chemotherapy, would, when Secretary of State for Northern Ireland, slam her wig down on the conference table to emphasise a point.

Neither long nor short, and in its way looking more like a wig than natural hair, was the short-lived and unattractively named 'ape' hairstyle that flourished briefly in the 1970s. It deserved a longer life, if only because it combined the charms of the long and the

FIG. 119. It was modern hair lacquers that made this 1960s style feasible. More sculpture than hairstyle – is it real or is it a wig? (photo Barnaby's Picture Library, London)

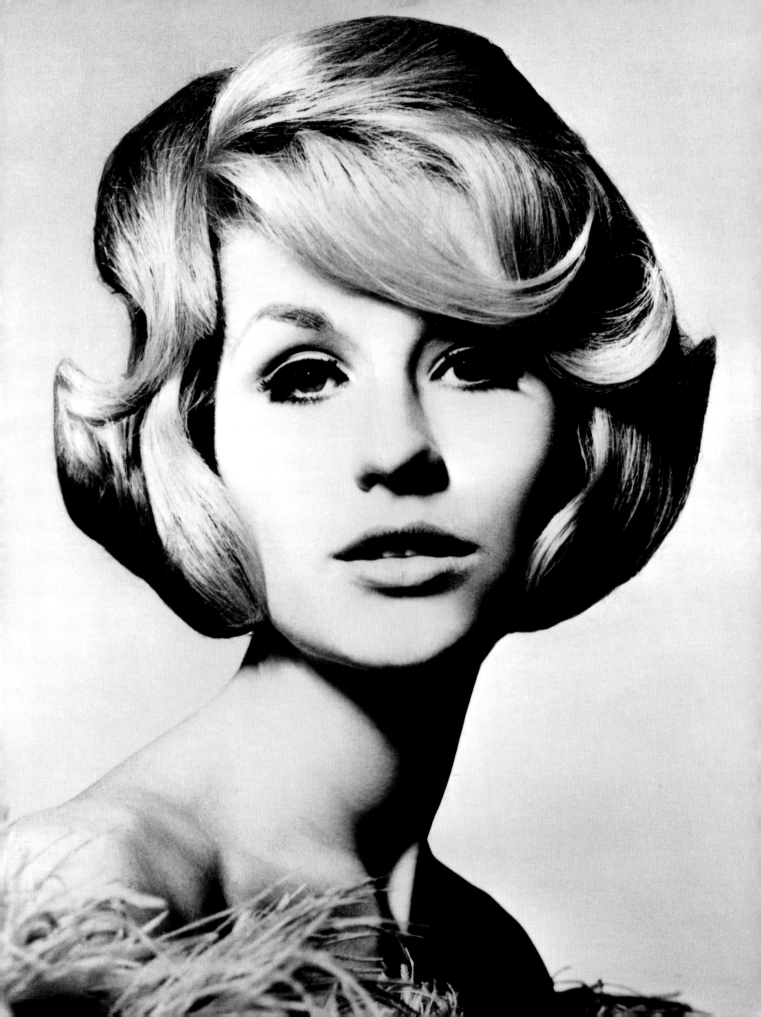

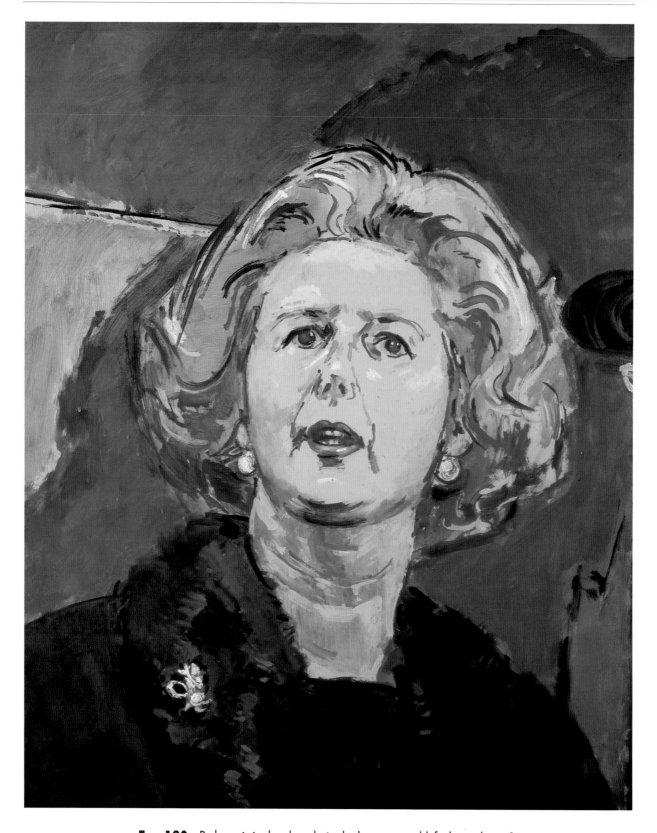

FIG. 120. Perhaps it is the short-haired who appear old-fashioned now?
Ruskin Spear, True Blue, Portrait of Margaret Thatcher, 1980s (Philip Mould Historical Portraits Ltd, London)

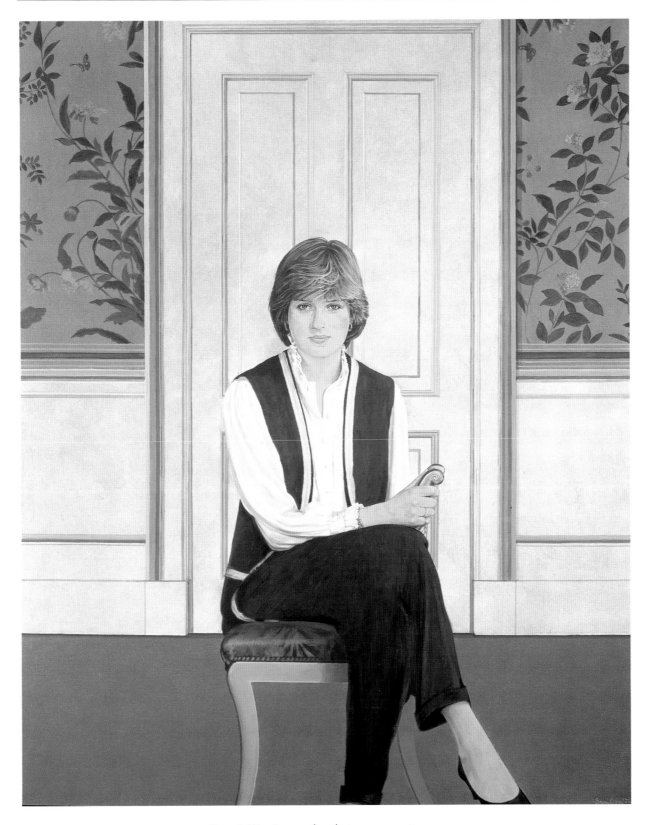

Fig. 121. A page-boy haircut on a princess.
Bryan Organ, *Diana, Princess of Wales*, 1981 (National Portrait Gallery, London)

because it combined the charms of the long and the short. The head would be closely cropped, usually with clustered curls, while the back could be as long as the wearer chose to grow it. It combined an eighteenth-century flavour with a twentieth-century practicality and an early version of it can indeed be seen in fig. 115, second from left.

Perhaps the 'ape' was a natural stepping stone to the reversal of the trend for short hair, in recent years, towards a return to an almost Victorian delight in relatively complex ways of wearing long hair. Possibly as a reaction to her mother's short hair and the way that she, as a child, likewise had her hair kept short, the

Jacqueline Du Pré will be remembered for her long blonde hair, rivalling in length the hair on her cello's bow

Princess Royal is today a 'real' princess, with long hair. She does not wear it hanging free like a medieval princess perhaps, but, more appropriately, she wears it as her crowning glory, befitting someone of the blood royal. It is also reminiscent of her grandmother and queens and princesses down the centuries. Nor is she alone in this comeback of the long-haired. Jacqueline Du Pré will be remembered for her long blonde hair, rivalling in length the hair on her cello's bow. Before her, a concert soloist would either have had short hair or hair carefully put up. The only exception would be those playing the harp and seeking a suitably Celtic or medieval image. Wearing her hair up was not Jacqueline Du Pré's style. However, it is now something that the long-haired can easily do and at will, with the help of simple, inexpensive devices such as large plastic claws – miniature versions of the old gin trap.

The social constraints are gone now, and, ironically, it is not necessarily the long-haired who appear formal and old-fashioned but the short-haired such as Mrs Thatcher (as she then was) in fig. 120. Her hair is almost wire-like in its forceful but feminine no-nonsense fashion. She owes as much to the availability of suitable sprays as her antithesis, a young man with a spiky punk style.

One must come finally to Diana, 'the people's princess'. In fig. 121 her eyes look out from under a heavy brow of hair, moulded over her ears like that of a medieval page or – more obviously – the Beatles, who rocketed to stardom when she was still a baby. She is gone now, but, clearly, such a simple haircut will prevail, whether for women or men. Diana's hairstyle is evidence that, although hair has a beauty all its own, a beautiful woman need not depend upon it as a major part of her armoury. It is evidence, too, of the return of the patrician as an arbiter of style. Who would have thought that checkout girls in supermarkets, who a quarter of a century before would have emulated pop singers from Liverpool, would, in the 1980s and '90s, aspire instead to copy the hairstyle of a Princess of Wales?

Revealingly, perhaps, it was Tony Blair who dubbed Diana 'the people's princess' after her death. In truth, however, she was the quintessential Sloane Ranger rather than one of the people, even to the extent of having taught in a nursery school not far from Sloane Square. So it was that, in the 1980s, Sloane Ranger mothers would forswear their shoulder-length hair and Alice bands in favour of a shorter 'Princess Di' style, ideally by Kevin Shanley at Headlines. They would, however, allow a rebellious 'Sloane' daughter to have a spiky post-punk cut by Sissors or Smile, as the Sloane Ranger Handbook of 1982 so meticulously tells us.

Now, in the post-Diana years, at the turn of the millennium, it is Cherie Blair and Hillary Clinton, on either side of the Atlantic, who carry the torch for the fashionably short-haired. Following in Diana's wake, they find to their cost that the casual hairstyle of a modern 'princess' can be very expensive to maintain, or so their hairdressers would have them believe. Indeed, these artists have them so much in thrall that no overseas official visit can be contemplated without them being part of the entourage – and the same goes for the

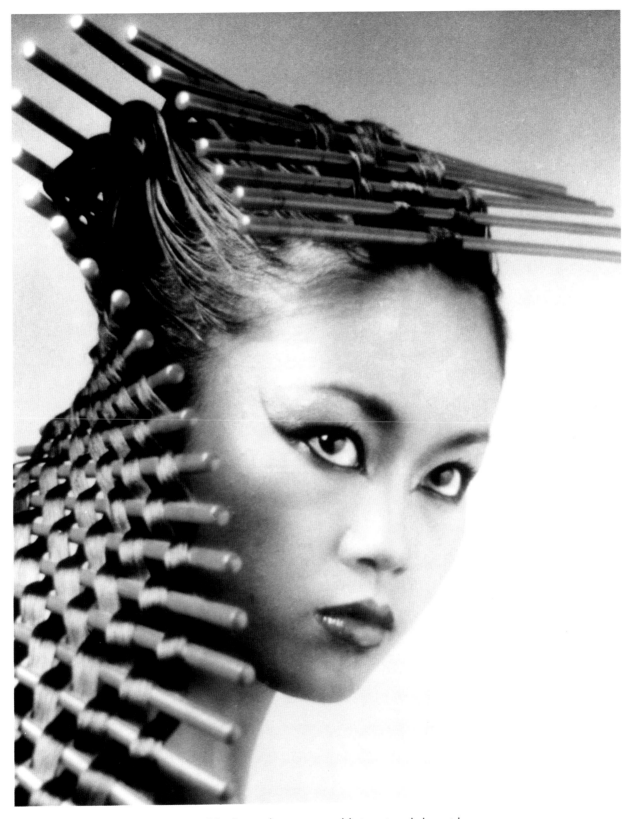

FIG. 122. Oriental eyes, oriental hair, oriental chopsticks
— all fused together in an exciting new composition. Hair by Soh (Camera Press)

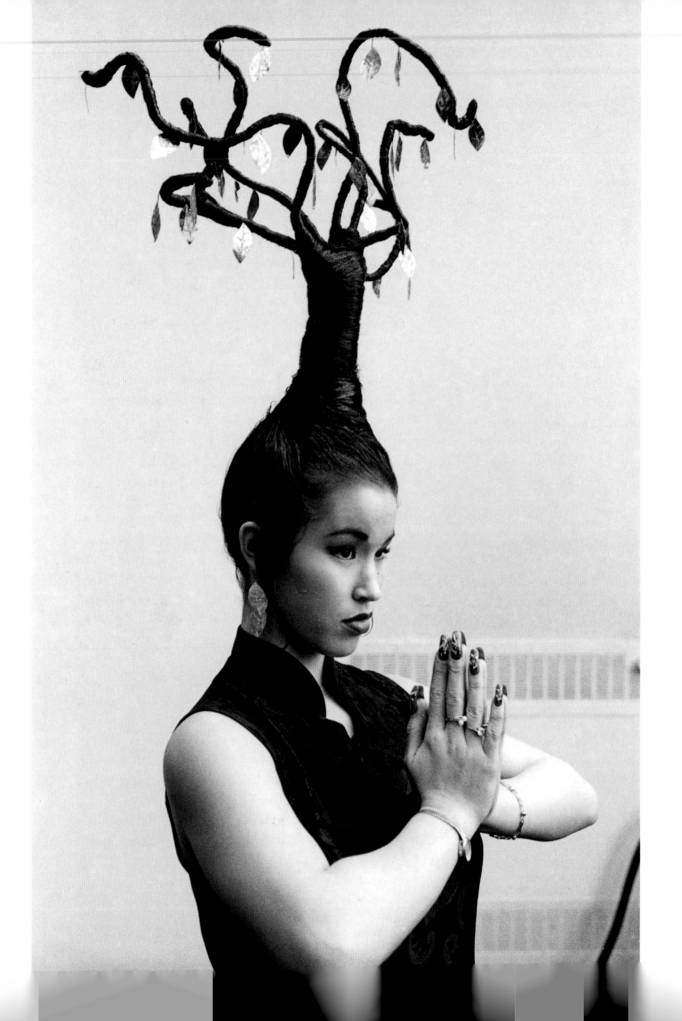

these haircuts are of legendary proportions, so as to make mere mortals wonder if the 'princess's haircut' is not as mythical as the 'emperor's new clothes' of the fairytale.

Equally legendary are the fees commanded by the fashion models of this world, Naomi Campbell and her ilk. In recent years, old-fashioned men have heaved a sigh of delight as they have watched them strutting their way down the catwalks with breathtakingly long hair swinging towards their buttocks – the antithesis of Cherie, Hillary and Diana.

Some of that frisson of delight, however, is diminished when it appears that much of this hair is no more than extensions, the latest development. These are not the wigs of the 1960s nor the transformations of the 1930s, but part of a new technology by which the short-haired can have long hair added to their own, and wash and treat it as if it was indeed their own. Time-consuming, expensive and short-lived though it be, it provides a realism that is unsurpassed in the whole history of hair.

However, wherever there is realism there is also the urge to create the unashamedly artificial, drawing liberally on a variety of cultures, freely adapted. One such is a creation by Soh (fig. 122) in which long oriental hair is woven round chopsticks, creating what amounts to a wattle fence down the girl's back. Equally arresting is the fantastic tree emerging from an upthrusting column of hair, putting one in mind of something on a willow pattern plate (fig. 123). Its chinoiserie is, though, no more Chinese than Wedgwood, this being a student exhibit at Croydon in 1997. But then, what is fashion without fantasy?

What will become popular as we progress further into the new millennium? Over the centuries hair has ranged through the full spectrum of styles, many seen repeatedly. That spectrum has expanded in recent years in response to new technology. However, even though, with extensions, the short-haired can become amazingly long-haired overnight, there will always be those who want to grow their own hair long and those who will suddenly tire of it.

The end of the twentieth century saw an age of tolerance about the way hair is worn. It is astonishing to record that, as recently as 1961, the land of the relatively long-haired Abraham Lincoln and Thomas Jefferson was actually throwing young men into prison because their hair was too long. Indeed, certain American states erected large hoardings along the roadsides urging: 'Keep America beautiful, get a haircut'. Now a woman may wear her hair as long or short as she likes, or have none at all, and a man may do likewise. There remain exceptions in a very few walks of life, but even then it is possible to sue employers for discrimination or wrongful dismissal. Nonetheless, as Ted Polhemus mooted and we discussed in opening, hair and the way it is worn does, and doubtless always will, remain something of a tribal distinguishing mark. However, it was Mrs Thatcher who insisted upon the importance of the individual. If someone decided to walk around like William the Conqueror, with the back of his head shaved, that would be his affair and few would question it, certainly not in the Western world. There comes a point when a tribal distinction is adopted by no more than a 'tribe' of one.

Desmond Morris pointed out in *The Naked Ape* that it is remarkable that we have hair at all, since we have such little use for it, other than decoratively. We may find, in time, that we no longer have it – evolution being what it is. That being the case, let us all continue to cherish our hair, its charms and its decorative potential. While some of us may lose our hair in the course of life, mankind itself may not have hair for many millennia more. Let us make the most of it while we can.

FIG. 123. Tree of Life? An experimental design at a students' exhibition, not in Kowloon but at the Fairfield Hall in Croydon, at the College Hair Styles Show of 1997. (Barnaby's Picture Library, London)

PHOTOGRAPHIC ACKNOWLEDGEMENTS

The publishers have made their best endeavours to trace all copyright holders but should there be any omissions we would be grateful to be informed.

Fig 1. Bridgeman Art Library
Fig. 2 Author
Fig. 3. Bridgeman Art Library
Fig. 4 Bridgeman Art Library
Fig. 5 Bridgeman Art Library
Fig. 6 Bridgeman Art Library
Fig. 7 Bridgeman Art Library
Fig. 8 Bridgeman Art Library
Fig. 9 Bridgeman Art Library
Fig. 10 British Museum
Fig. 11 British Museum
Fig. 12 British Museum
Fig. 13 British Museum
Fig. 14 Bridgeman Art Library
Fig. 15 British Museum
Fig. 16 British Museum
Fig. 17 Bridgeman Art Library
Fig. 18 British Museum
Fig. 19 Bridgeman Art Library
Fig. 20 Bridgeman Art Library
Fig. 21 Bridgeman Art Library
Fig. 22 Bridgeman Art Library
Fig. 23 Bridgeman Art Library
Fig. 24 Bridgeman Art Library
Fig. 25 Bridgeman Art Library
Fig. 26 Bridgeman Art Library
Fig. 27 Bridgeman Art Library
Fig. 28 Bridgeman Art Library
Fig. 29 Bridgeman Art Library
Fig. 30 Bridgeman Art Library
Fig. 31 Bridgeman Art Library
Fig. 32 Bridgeman Art Library
Fig. 33 © National Gallery, London
Fig. 34 Bridgeman Art Library
Fig. 35 © National Portrait Gallery, London
Fig. 36 Author
Fig. 37 Bridgeman Art Library
Fig. 38 Author
Fig. 39 Author

Fig. 40 © National Portrait Gallery, London
Fig. 41 © National Portrait Gallery, London
Fig. 42 © National Portrait Gallery, London
Fig. 43 Author
Fig. 44 Birmingham City Council
Fig. 45 Bridgeman Art Library
Fig. 46 Bridgeman Art Library
Fig. 47 Bridgeman Art Library
Fig. 48 Bridgeman Art Library
Fig. 49 Bridgeman Art Library
Fig. 50 Bridgeman At Library
Fig. 51 Bridgeman Art Library
Fig. 52 Bridgeman Art Library
Fig. 53 Bridgeman Art Library
Fig. 54 Author
Fig. 55 Author
Fig. 56 Author
Fig. 57 Bridgeman Art Library
Fig. 58 Bridgeman Art Library
Fig. 59 Bridgeman Art Library
Fig. 60 Bridgeman Art Library
Fig. 61 Bridgeman Art Library
Fig. 62 Bridgeman Art Library
Fig. 63 Bridgeman Art Library
Fig. 64 Bridgeman Art Library
Fig. 65 Bridgeman Art Library
Fig. 66 © National Portrait Gallery, London
Fig. 67 © National Portrait Gallery, London
Fig. 68 Bridgeman Art Library
Fig. 69 Bridgeman Art Library
Fig. 70 Bridgeman Art Library
Fig. 71 Author
Fig. 72 Author
Fig. 73 © National Portrait Gallery, London
Fig. 74 © National Portrait Gallery, London
Fig. 75 Author
Fig. 76 Bridgeman Art Library
Fig. 77 Bridgeman Art Library
Fig. 78 Bridgeman Art Library
Fig. 79 The Hirschsprung Collection, Copenhagen

Fig. 80 Bridgeman Art Library
Fig. 81 © National Portrait Gallery, London
Fig. 82 Bridgeman Art Library
Fig. 83 Bridgeman Art Library
Fig. 84 Dodge & Sons, Sherborne
Fig. 85 Bridgeman Art Library
Fig. 86 Bridgeman Art Library
Fig. 87 Bridgeman Art Library
Fig. 88 Bridgeman Art Library
Fig. 89 Museum of Fine Art Boston
Fig 90 Bridgeman Art Library
Fig. 92 © National Portrait Gallery, London
Fig. 93 Author
Fig. 94 Bridgeman Art Library
Fig. 95 Author
Fig. 96 Author
Fig. 97 Author
Fig. 98 Author
Fig. 99 Bridgeman Art Library
Fig. 100 Bridgeman Art Library
Fig. 105 Bridgeman Art Library
Fig. 106 Author
Fig. 107 Author
Fig. 108 Bridgeman Art Library
Fig. 109 Bridgeman Art Library
Fig. 110 © National Portrait Gallery, London
Fig. 111 Bridgeman Art Library
Fig. 112 © Lewis Morley/Akehurst Bureau courtesy National Portrait Gallery, London
Fig. 113 Aquarius
Fig 114 Universal Pictorial Press and Agency Ltd
Fig. 115 UA/CIP courtesy Aquarius
Fig. 116 Hulton Getty Picture Gallery
Fig. 117 Richard Lines, Ringwood
Fig. 118 Chris Wroblewski Skin Shows, London
Fig. 119 Barnaby's Picture Library
Fig. 120 Bridgeman Art Library
Fig. 121 © National Portrait Gallery, London
Fig. 122 Camera Press
Fig. 123 Barnaby's Picture Library